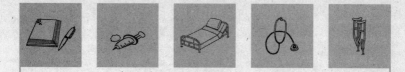

HOW TO SURVIVE YOUR HOSPITAL STAY

The Complete Guide to Getting the Care You Need—

and Avoiding Problems You Don't

Gail Van Kanegan, R.N., M.S.N., C.N.P.,
and
Michael Boyette

A Lynn Sonberg Book

A Fireside Book / Published by Simon & Schuster
New York   London   Toronto   Sydney   Singapore

FIRESIDE
Rockefeller Center
1230 Avenue of the Americas
New York, NY 10020

FIRESIDE and colophon are registered trademarks
of Simon & Schuster, Inc.

For information regarding special discounts for bulk purchases, please
contact Simon & Schuster Special Sales at 1-800-456-6798 or
business@simonandschuster.com

A Lynn Sonberg Book

Designed by William Ruoto

Manufactured in the United States of America
10 9 8 7 6 5 4 3 2 1

Library of Congress Cataloging-in-Publication Data
Van Kanegan, Gail.
How to survive your hospital stay : the complete guide to getting the
care you need—and avoiding the problems you don't / Gail Van
Kanegan and Michael Boyette.
p. cm.
"A Lynn Sonberg book."
"A Fireside book."
Includes bibliographical references and index.
1. Hospital patients. 2. Hospital care. 3. Consumer education. I.
Michael Boyette. II. Title.

ISBN 0-7432-3319-0

Disclaimer

This publication contains the opinions and ideas of its authors. It is intended to provide helpful and informative material on the subjects addressed in the publication. It is sold with the understanding that the authors and publisher are not engaged in rendering medical, health, or any other kind of personal professional services in the book. The reader should consult his or her medical, health, or other competent professional before adopting any of the suggestions in this book or drawing inferences from it.

The authors and publisher specifically disclaim all responsibility for any liability, loss, or risk, personal or otherwise, which is incurred as a consequence, directly or indirectly, of the use and application of any of the contents of this book.

CONTENTS

Preface

This book is an essential guide for anyone who ever expects to be admitted to a hospital, or who has a loved one going into a hospital—in other words, just about everyone, sooner or later. It offers simple ideas that can help patients and their families avoid hospital hazards and substandard care.

Both of us, Gail Van Kanegan and Michael Boyette, have spent a lot of time grappling with issues of hospital safety. Gail is a registered nurse who's worked in just about every clinical department at hospitals. She later went on to become a certified advanced practice nurse, a nurse specialist with a master's degree in nursing. Today, she works as a family nurse practitioner, with a focus on patient education and prevention of disease. Over the years, Gail's seen firsthand many of the problems we discuss in this book, and she's seen how important it is for patients to understand what's happening and take charge of their hospital care.

Michael Boyette is a longtime medical journalist with roots in the hospital world too. In the early 1980s, he covered the emerging field of risk management. Hospitals were facing a crisis of rising malpractice claims and were looking for ways to reduce their risk and avoid lawsuits. As editor of a publication for hospital risk managers, he interviewed hundreds of experts on malpractice and countless practitioners from the front lines of hospitals. He quickly discovered that lawsuits were just a symptom of a deeper problem: At the time, hospitals did a bad job of identifying and preventing problems that put patients at risk. Many doctors, nurses, and administrators assumed that these risks were an inevitable part of modern medicine. Since then, they've learned otherwise, and they've become much better at controlling these risks.

From both our backgrounds, we've learned one compelling fact: *An educated patient is the best protection against medical errors.* Hospitals have invested billions of dollars in trying to create systems that will keep patients safe. In many cases, these efforts have been successful—to cite just one example, blood-infection rates in hospitals have declined between 31 and 43 percent in intensive care units since 1990. But they still need your help to help you get better.

Patients and their families often feel like David against health care Goliaths. All that technology, all that knowledge, all those experts, all that money! Who's going to listen to a mere patient?

Yet we've seen time and again that patients are often a major catalyst for change. Consider the impact, for example, that expecting mothers had on obstetrics. Most of the innovations we now take for granted—birthing suites, fathers in the delivery room, less reliance on drugs, natural childbirth, to name a few—came about because patients and families got involved in making decisions about their health care. We treat mental illness more effectively than ever before—in part because patients and their families became active partners in their care. And today, doctors and hospitals take a more compassionate and patient-centered approach to end-of-life treatment. We have innovations such as hospice care and living wills because terminal patients and families insisted on being treated with greater dignity and respect.

Doctors' attitudes have changed profoundly in the decades since we first became involved in health care. Twenty and thirty years ago, most doctors resented patients who did their own independent research, looked into alternatives the doctor hadn't mentioned, and showed up at the office with a long list of technical questions about their treatment. Today, doctors expect that degree of patient involvement—and the best doctors welcome it.

It is our hope that this book will contribute in some small way to a similar revolution in patient safety. Hospitals, medical schools, government agencies, and research organizations have made vast efforts to find ways to make hospitals safer. But they can't do it alone. Choose to be an active partner in your hospital care. It's good for your health—and for the health of the hospital.

Acknowledgments

Although I am a longtime veteran of nursing, this is my first book, and a number of people have helped me with it. I would like to thank Barb Bancroft, a fellow nurse practitioner and colleague from CPP Associates, for having the vision and confidence that I could do this. *How to Survive Your Hospital Stay* would not be a reality without Barb's influence, confidence, and friendship. Barb, thank you.

Without research, progress is not possible. I give thanks to Arlis Dittmer, M.A.L.S., from Blessing-Rieman College of Nursing. She and her staff assisted with obtaining numerous articles and guided me through much of the research needed for this book.

My nursing colleagues provided important information on current hospital standards of care. Cathy Aschemann, R.N., B.S.N., accepted my calls at all hours of the day or night to answer my questions and redirect my thoughts. Thank you for your professional assistance and for the years of our friendship.

I would like to thank Michael Boyette, my coauthor, for his expertise in journalism and his guidance throughout the writing process. I would not have been capable of pulling all of the information together without him. Michael edited my work over and over until I got it right and made my ideas flow for others to understand. Michael, I am grateful for your assistance and guidance.

To Lynn Sonberg, of Lynn Sonberg Book Associates, I thank you for your willingness to take a chance with me. I am grateful that you have compassion for hospital patients, current and future. Your caring will bring better health to a world of people.

I feel that all patients and their families need to be thanked for sharing the life experiences that make this book unique. In the thirty years that I have been in nursing, I have experienced and witnessed how people heal and how complications from illness can stop that process. My own experiences as a patient have also given me a better understanding of how it feels to be helpless and dependent on others. This has shaped my approach to nursing. I am also acutely aware of how little knowledge the communities we live in have about their rights to health care. Being a patient advocate was one of the first things I learned in nursing school. I thank all of my instructors and mentors through the years who have helped shape my approach to nursing.

Gail Van Kanegan

Introduction

Keeping Yourself Safe

If you or someone you love is going into a hospital, you need this book.

Most hospitals work hard to make sure you get the care you need and to protect you from harm. And most doctors and nurses are dedicated, competent professionals, committed to helping you heal. But the modern hospital is a vast, complex enterprise, and there are many opportunities for things to go wrong. The best way to protect yourself is to be an informed consumer.

Reliable estimates suggest that, of every one hundred people who go into a hospital, between five and ten will suffer some sort of injury or complication as a result.

Consider these statistics:

- The *Los Angeles Times* reports that as many as 180,000 Americans may be killed each year by injuries, hospital infections, misdiagnosis, mishandling, and other avoidable hospital-related fatalities. That's as many people as would be killed if a jumbo jet crashed every day of the year.

- The Centers for Disease Control estimates that about two million people contract hospital infections in the United States each year—more than one in twenty hospitalized patients. About eighty thousand people die as a result. That means hospital infections alone rank as the fourth most common cause of death in America, killing more people than auto accidents and homicides combined.

- A 1998 study published in *The Journal of the American Medical Association* estimated that one hundred thousand Americans die in hospitals each year from adverse drug reactions.

- The Centers for Disease Control estimates that as many as sixty million antibiotic prescriptions written each year are unnecessary and potentially dangerous.

- According to the *Detroit News,* "one of every five patients who died in the medical intensive care unit at one of the nation's best hospitals was misdiagnosed" by his or her doctor.

Keep in mind that we're not talking here about treatment *failures*—people who go into a hospital and don't get better. We're talking about *new* injuries and diseases that people suffer as a *direct result* of their hospital care: infections they didn't have when they went in, receiving the wrong medications, poor nutrition, misdiagnosis.

Nor are we talking about *inevitable* complications, such as a surgeon performing a delicate operation and damaging nearby organs. Most hospital illnesses and injuries are preventable by following simple principles of good care—things like nurses and technicians washing their hands between patients, using simple checklists to avoid medication errors, or writing instructions legibly.

Now the good news:

Armed with the knowledge in this book, *you and your loved ones have the power to avoid most of these risks.*

Hospitals and health care researchers have invested millions—perhaps billions—of dollars to discover what the greatest risks are and how they can be prevented.

By and large, the problem isn't with exotic equipment or new experimental treatments. It's the everyday stuff. People in a hurry. Or not paying attention because they've done something a thousand times before. Or making assumptions without double-checking. And it's often the same kinds of errors, happening time and time again, that cause the most harm.

You Can Protect Yourself

Of course, hospitals try very hard not to make mistakes and to head off problems. But in any large organization, with so many people doing so many different things, something is bound to go wrong.

That's where you and your family have an advantage.

You don't have to worry about running the whole hospital, or taking care of hundreds of sick patients. You have to worry only about you.

Armed with the right information, you and your family are the best protection against hospital-related injuries and illness.

That's the purpose of this book—to arm you with the information you need, in an easy-to-use format.

When you or your loved one is going into a hospital,

you don't have time to wade through a lot of research. Nor can we discuss every conceivable risk in hospitals. Some risks are relatively rare and hard to defend against. There are other risks that, frankly, you don't have much control over.

But it is possible for you to protect yourself against most of the serious risks that you'll encounter in the hospital. We've identified the ten most serious you'll face during your hospital stay. For each, we offer *simple, practical steps* you can take before, during, and after your stay to protect yourself or your loved one from harm.

Focus on these, and you will emerge from the hospital in better health and better prepared for your recovery.

In the pages that follow, we offer you a series of practical steps that:

- show what you can do before you're admitted to the hospital
- identify and avoid the top ten risks while you're hospitalized
- explain what to do when you're ready to be discharged to keep you healthy at home and avoid later complications

Keep this guide close at hand. Refer to it often. Whether this is your first time dealing with hospitals or you're an old hand, you'll find useful suggestions and ideas that will help you come home healthy.

How to Use This Book

In the pages that follow, we identify practical strategies that can help you remain healthy and avoid risks during your hospital stay. You don't need to be a medical expert to follow them, and they won't in any way interfere with the course of treatment that your doctor has prescribed. Indeed, we urge you to review them with your doctor and seek his or her input.

Most suggestions are based on common sense, because that's the best way to stay out of trouble. Most involve making sure that people do what they already know they're supposed to do. Most medical errors occur not because of ignorance but due to neglect. Hospitals are busy, complicated places, often running shorthanded and under difficult cost constraints. If you know what to look for, you can do a lot to head off problems.

Your most important tool in this effort is a pleasant but firm attitude. Treat your caregivers with respect and insist on respect in return.

We recognize, of course, that it may be hard to be proactive when you're headed for the hospital. You may be in pain. You may be weak or disoriented. Perhaps you're scared. You'll certainly have a lot on your mind already. That's why we suggest that it's best to find a trusted friend or family member who can act as your advocate and help you take the necessary steps.

But even if you don't have an advocate, you can benefit from the ideas in this book. Especially in Part 2, we focus on steps you can take yourself—from your own hospital bed—to help ensure your safety. Often it's a matter of asking the right questions—repeatedly, if necessary—until you get the information you need to make good decisions. Other times, it's simply reminding your caregivers of things they already know and encouraging them to stop and think before acting.

By and large, the care you receive in the hospital will probably be competent and professional. Many patients go through their entire hospital stay without being exposed to medical mistakes or undue risks. And we aren't suggesting that you or your advocate has to be on guard twenty-four hours a day. Rather, our aim is to alert you to red flags, so that you can focus your (sometimes) limited energies where they can really make a difference.

You may not be willing or able to follow every recommendation we make here. It depends on your individual circumstances—why you're going into the hospital, how long you'll be there, and what happens while you're there. It also depends on what you're comfortable with. Do as much as you can. Every step you take will help you be that much safer.

A couple of housekeeping notes: Though this book is a collaboration, it's written in one voice—Gail's—for the sake of simplicity. Similarly, we address the book to you, the patient, for reasons of simplicity and readability. But we're really speaking to your loved ones too. When patients are seriously ill, it often falls to others to look out for their interests. In those circumstances, all of the recommendations we offer can be followed by your family, loved ones, or advocate.

HOW TO
SURVIVE YOUR
HOSPITAL STAY

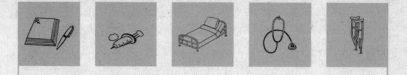

PART ONE

Eight Important Ways to Prepare for Your Hospital Stay

A safe hospital stay begins before you're admitted. If you think you might have to go into the hospital anytime soon, start making preparations early. Even if you don't have much time before you go, you and your loved ones can make some key decisions quickly that can have a big effect on your health. For example, you can spend about a half hour on one Web site (see Chapter 6) and get detailed information that allows you to compare hospitals in your area. You can prepare yourself mentally as well, because if you enter the hospital with the right mind-set, you'll be much safer.

In this section, we offer eight simple strategies that will fully prepare you for your hospital visit.

1

Avoid the Hospital—if You Can

One of the best ways to avoid the dangers in hospitals is to stay out of the hospital. But if you must go, ask your doctor what can be done to keep your stay there as short as possible.

That may sound like strange advice. After all, nobody *wants* to go into a hospital. People go into the hospital only because they have to, right?

Well, the reality is a bit more complicated. Over the past twenty years, we've learned that many traditional hospital services can be delivered just as effectively to outpatients. Many types of surgery, imaging services (such as X rays and CT scans), and even childbirth are now offered on an outpatient basis.

Equally important, we've learned that hospital stays can be reduced dramatically. For example, patients can complete much of their recovery at home, under the care of home health nurses, or in "step-down" units that are separate from the hospital. And driven by cost considerations, hospitals have become more efficient about scheduling tests and procedures.

The reason? Money. Insurance companies want you to stay out of those expensive hospitals if possible. And if you have to go in, they want to rush you through as quickly as possible to avoid racking up huge bills.

The hospital has a similar incentive. In the old days, hospitals were mostly paid by the day—so the longer you stayed, the more they could bill your insurance company. These days, they're more likely to be paid by the diagnosis. If you go into the hospital for, say, a hernia operation, the surgeon and hospital receive a fixed payment, whether you're in for one day or two weeks. So the hospital will do its best to get you in and out quickly, all in an effort to free up your bed for the next paying patient.

It's true that hospitals' move-'em-through approach can make you feel like you're on a medical assembly line. But though their motives may be crass, they're often doing you a favor—because *the less time you spend in a hospital, the fewer opportunities arise for things to go wrong.* The situation is exactly like driving. Your car insurance company can give you a better rate if you don't drive as much, because you're less likely to get in an accident when your car is sitting in your driveway.

Consumer groups often miss the point on this issue. They assume that *more* hospital care is *better* care. In 1996, for example, Congress passed legislation mandating that health plans pay for minimum hospital stays for new mothers. Many new mothers complained about being forced out of hospitals when they were barely recovered from a cesarean section or difficult birth. Hearings exposed horror stories of sick infants sent home too soon, only to be rushed back to the emergency room because of life-threatening complications. Politicians called the practice "drive-by deliveries."

Some of these mothers shouldn't have been sent home so soon, of course. Some needed monitoring or treatment. But the idea that *all* new mothers benefit from a mandated minimum stay is wrong. All things being equal, healthy mothers and infants are much safer at home than at the hospital—even if being home is more difficult or uncomfortable. They face less chance of exposure to infection, especially the drug-resistant infections that flourish in hospitals. Less chance of getting the wrong medication. Less chance of somebody making a mistake.

Of course, nobody should be sent home from the hospital too soon, especially not just because a health plan is trying to cut corners. But mandating longer hospital stays makes about as much sense as forcing children to play in the middle of a busy street.

The same goes for anyone in the hospital. If you're there because you need hospital care, that's one thing. But if you're staying an extra day or two because of a scheduling problem with one of your tests, or because the doctor is on vacation, or because the hospital is trying to get more money out of your insurance company, you're at unnecessary risk. And if your insurance plan would rather you were discharged and have the tests done later as an outpatient, you might be better off, even if it is an inconvenience.

Strategies for Avoiding a Hospital Stay

Talk to your doctor. The best way to avoid a hospital stay is to tell your doctor what you want. Sometimes a doctor will recommend a hospital stay because it's more convenient than outpatient care—especially if you need a series of tests, or if you require home care. If you'd rather put up with inconvenience and stay out of the hospital, tell the doctor; that is one of your rights to health care.

Find out whether you're a good candidate for outpatient care. Discuss it with your doctor. Some considerations include your overall health (the healthier you are, the quicker you'll recover), your support system (do you have family or friends who can help you?), your ability to follow directions and perform any necessary aftercare, and, of course, the type of tests or procedures you need.

Ask your doctor whether any hospital tests or procedures can be done before you go in or after you're discharged. The more you can have done as an outpatient, the less time you need to spend in the hospital. Also, you don't have to lie around simply waiting for test results to come back.

Plan ahead. Before you go in, look into home care and aftercare options. You may be able to get discharged sooner if these arrangements are in place.

Know what procedures can be done as an outpatient. About 75 to 80 percent of all operations, procedures, and tests can be performed in a same-day surgery center. Find out what's available in your area. Here are some typical procedures:

- dermatologic procedures, including most types of plastic surgery
- knee and shoulder repair, up to and including joint replacements
- hernia repair
- gallbladder removal
- diagnostic procedures such as cystoscopy, endoscopy, and colonoscopy
- biopsy: lung, breast, liver, stomach
- removal of some tumors, depending on their location
- gynecologic procedures, such as D&Cs and laparoscopic tubal ligations
- childbirth
- sinus surgery and other ear, nose, and throat procedures
- myelograms for diagnosing back pain
- cardiac procedures, including cardiac catheterizations and cardioversions (conversions of abnormal heartbeats)
- arteriograms to diagnose problems in the arteries
- blood transfusions
- intravenous therapy
- surgery of the eye
- oral surgery, including wisdom tooth extractions

Find an accredited facility. The Accreditation Association for Ambulatory Health Care evaluates day surgery programs. You can check credentials on its Web site at www.aaahc.org.

2

Choose a Health Care Advocate

We asked doctors and nurses, "If you were going into the hospital right now, what's the first thing you would do?"

Just about every one said the same thing: Choose a health care advocate.

Whether you're going into the hospital several weeks from now for elective surgery, or you're sitting in the emergency room right now waiting to be admitted, your most important first step is selecting someone you trust to be your health care advocate before and during your stay.

The reason: From the moment you're admitted, you lose a great deal of your ability to exert control over your own care. No matter how accomplished or powerful you are in your own world, in the hospital you are a *patient*— dependent on the hospital for your most basic needs.

In theory, of course, you're still in charge of your health care. You give up none of your rights when you enter a hospital and turn in your street clothes for that oversized bib they call a gown. Legally, nobody can force you to take the pills they bring you, submit to all those needles and IV lines, put up with the endless tests and procedures. Technically, you're free to get up and walk out if you don't like the service you're getting.

Of course, therein lies the problem. You aren't really in a position to do any of those things. For all practical purposes, you're dependent on the hospital and the staff. You need the treatment they offer, or you wouldn't be there. Chances are, you're not feeling so great either. And the last thing someone in that position of dependency wants to do is buck the system or anger the people who have so much control over your well-being.

And yet, as we've pointed out, your well-being often *requires* someone to challenge—or at least confront—the system. Someone who can speak from a position of strength and independence. A health care advocate.

A health care advocate in this sense doesn't necessarily mean a lawyer or legal guardian. Nor does it mean someone who's going to take a confrontational position. It's simply someone who is able and willing to act on your behalf while you're in the hospital—a single point of contact who will represent you and look out for your interests during the hospitalization. It may be your spouse, your child, another relative, even a friend. Your health care advocate does not have to be your selected Power of Attorney for health care, as described in Chapter 8.

Be careful, by the way, not to confuse this role with a so-called patient advocate that many hospitals have on their staffs. That position is really a sort of ombudsman or problem solver, whose job is to respond to patients' problems or complaints. Such a person may be quite useful in helping you cut through red tape or get answers to your questions, but in the final analysis you need an advocate who works for you, not for the hospital.

The most important attribute for your health care advocate is the willingness and ability to *speak up*—to ask questions when things happen that you don't understand and to insist that people take the necessary measures to protect you from harm.

The ideal health care advocate is also:

Medically knowledgeable, able to speak the language of health care. If you have a friend or relative who's a nurse, a physician, a medical technician, or even a medical secretary, think about asking him or her to serve as your advocate—or to help your health care advocate understand what's going on from a medical standpoint. This person doesn't need to have any special expertise in your disease or condition; most important is the ability to ask the right questions and understand the hospital jargon.

Assertive but not aggressive. Look for someone who's able to get things done without making people mad, someone who has a knack for being persistent but polite. The last thing you want is for your health care advocate to create a crisis. A good advocate keeps his or her eye on the ultimate goal—protecting your health and safety—and does whatever it takes to ensure that goal.

Trustworthy. You may be literally trusting your life to your health care advocate, so you need someone you can count on. It's a big job to serve as someone's advocate, so be sure your advocate will see it through and that you can count on him or her to make good decisions.

Available. An effective health care advocate may have to spend several hours a day on your behalf at the beginning of your hospital stay and when you're getting ready to leave. He or she must have time to deal with doctors, nurses, and even family members, either on the phone or in person. He or she must have time to listen, ask questions, and deal with the hospital bureaucracy. Fortunately, most hospital stays are no more than a few days, but your advocate must understand the commitment that will be needed. If the job is too big, it's better to find out sooner rather than later, so you can make other arrangements.

Sometimes it might be possible to split the job among several people. If you do, be sure there's one point person who's clearly in charge and able to coordinate the effort. You don't want several people dealing with the doctor and hospital, asking the same questions and giving them conflicting information about your needs.

Familiar with any special fears or concerns, wishes or instructions you have about your hospital stay. For example, if you're scheduled for an MRI scan and you're concerned that you'll feel claustrophobic when you're put into the machine, your health care advocate should insist that you're sedated before the procedure. Make a list of your wishes.

Think about whether you want your health care advocate or someone else to make decisions if you become incapacitated or unable to make your wishes known. You need to make a living will to designate who will speak for you in such circumstances, as well as any special instructions for your care (see Chapter 8).

Your health care advocate may be the right person to

fulfill this role—but not necessarily. For example, you may want someone who's a little less close to the situation to be your health care advocate—a good friend or family member who can deal with the day-to-day issues during your hospital stay—and still have your spouse or significant other responsible for the big decisions.

Organized. Your health care advocate should be the point person for information related to your care. He or she should get copies of any information that you receive—for example, instructions for when you go home. Encourage your advocate to gather all this information in one place, such as a file folder or notebook, and keep it with him or her during your hospital stay.

If You Don't Have a Health Care Advocate

If you're not able to arrange for a health care advocate, don't despair. You can still take steps to ensure a safer hospital stay.

If the job is too big for any one person to take on, consider asking people to share it. For example, a friend who's a nurse may be able to help you understand your options but may not have the time or inclination to talk to your doctors. In this case, your friend in nursing can help you come up with the right questions to ask. Or you might have several family members take turns—a day or two each, for example, as long as you're hospitalized.

Often, your nurses can be effective health care advocates, especially if you make clear to them that you don't have family members or friends who can look out for your interests. Some nurses are better than others at listening to patients. Don't hesitate to share your questions or concerns with them and enlist their help, even if they're not your regular nurses.

And if necessary, you can act as your own advocate. Granted, that's not always so easy if you're seriously ill, in pain, sedated, or under a lot of stress. But even a modest effort can help. For example, simply by asking questions you prompt your caregivers to stop and think about what they're doing. And that, in and of itself, can go a long way toward keeping you safe.

Finally, remember that it doesn't have to be a full-time job. You don't need someone constantly looking over your caregivers' shoulders. There are certain critical periods during your hospital stay—when you're admitted, when you're discharged, and before any major procedure—when errors are most likely to occur. Get help for these times, and you're well on your way to a safe hospital stay.

3

Prepare Your Mind

In 1971, psychology professor Philip Zimbardo at Stanford University conducted an experiment with a group of college students. He randomly divided the group in half and assigned the first half to serve as "guards" and the second half to serve as "prisoners." He set up a "prison" in the basement of the psychology building and put the guards in charge. Then he filmed the interactions.

Even though the students knew that it was just an experiment, they quickly fell into their roles. The "guards" became officious, condescending, and intimidating. The "prisoners" became passive and withdrawn.

The experiment was supposed to last two weeks. Zimbardo canceled it after six days, worried that the guards were on the verge of physically abusing the prisoners.

The lesson? More than we care to think, the way we act is determined by external circumstances, giving us a role we happen to be playing at any given time.

That's just as true when you go into a hospital. You're not a prisoner, of course. And the people who work there aren't your guards. But many things about a hospital make patients feel powerless and passive: illness, pain, fear, lack of knowledge, the environment. When you enter a hospital, the first thing you do is surrender those things that represent your independence: your clothes, your valuables, your wallet and car keys. In their place, you get a thin, drafty gown and a hospital-issued ID bracelet. Often, you're hooked up to an infusion pump or other equipment that makes it difficult or impossible for you even to get up and take a walk. Your bed has bars on it. You don't even have your own space—usually, you're sharing a room with a stranger, and people you don't know walk in and out at all hours of the day and night.

Psychologically, that puts you in the same boat as those unfortunate college students. They weren't really prisoners either. They had the right to get up and walk out of the experiment whenever they wanted. Yet they didn't. Their sense of power and identity was diminished so quickly and so completely that they simply submitted to the harsh treatment.

This powerlessness puts you at risk in hospitals. Here's a real-life example:

A physician wrote an order for a patient who was having problems with his ears. On the order, the doctor wrote that the medication was to be dispensed "in r. ear"—that is, in the patient's right ear. (That's not how a prescription should be written, anyway, but that's another matter.) The doctor's handwriting was so bad that the letters ran together and the period was hardly visible (illegible prescriptions are another big problem). So the patient got his medication—you guessed it—"in rear."

While there was no major harm done except to the patient's dignity, this is a perfect illustration of how things go wrong in hospitals: A hurried physician writes an unclear order. An equally hurried nurse doesn't bother to check the patient's chart to see what his ailment was, or take the time to look up a medication she's unfamiliar with (if she had, she'd have known where it should have been administered).

But consider also how the patient's last and most important line of defense was breached: his own common sense. If his right ear hurt, why would he let someone turn him over and administer drops in his rectum? And when else in his life would he let someone do that without at least asking why? Why didn't he speak up?

Your best protection against medical mistakes is your right to say no. But it's hard to exercise that right when you're sick, worried, and stripped of the things that make you feel like a competent adult.

Strategies for Mental Preparation

It's important to maintain your sense of power and control in these circumstances. Here are some ideas that can help.

Recognize that you *will* feel powerless. People who always feel that they're in control of their lives are often surprised and overwhelmed by their feelings when they go into a hospital. It can be a disorienting and frightening experience. Remember that it's an extremely common reaction to hospitalization. And keep in mind that it's the *situation* that's making you feel that way, not some flaw or weakness on your part.

Maintain control over your person and environment— at least as much as you can. Little things matter a lot, because they serve as symbols of your independence and connect you with the rest of your life. Bring your own robe and slippers from home. Bring in pictures of your family, or whatever you need to remind you of your other roles in life.

Choose to be an *active* part of the team. Don't be passive. Ask questions if you don't understand something. Find out what's being done to you and why. You're not bothering anyone—most nurses and doctors prefer treating patients who are involved and interested in their care.

Be assertive but not combative. If you know your rights, you won't need to treat the staff with aggression or hostility. And recognize that a hospital is not a hotel. Don't use up all your energy (and goodwill with the staff) complaining about the food or the view from your window. Save your complaints for what's really important— for times when your health or safety is at stake.

Language to Win Over Your Health Care Team

Nurses and doctors are only human. If they feel attacked, they're likely to become defensive and resentful.

The right language can go a long way toward getting them to be more responsive to your needs. Consider this exchange:

NURSE: Okay, Mrs. Watson, we're going to send you down to radiology for some X rays. The orderly will be here in a few minutes.

PATIENT: I don't need any X rays. I had them taken a week ago, before I was admitted.

NURSE: Well, you'll have to take it up with your doctor. These orders are from the radiologist.

PATIENT: Doesn't he know I've already had X rays? Did he even bother to check?

NURSE: Ma'am, the radiologist will have to explain it to you. We just follow the orders. Besides, it's just a few X rays.

PATIENT: I don't need X rays. You people don't know what you're doing.

NURSE: Mrs. Watson, they're very busy down in radiology. If you don't go right now, you're going to be stuck down there until they can fit you in. That could take hours. It's up to you.

In this exchange, the patient assumes the role of expert ("I don't need X rays") and turns the exchange into an attack on the nurse's and hospital's competence. So it's no surprise that the nurse falls back on bureaucratic responses: "I'm only following orders." "You'll miss your place in line." The nurse has become more interested in defending her actions than in listening to the patient.

Instead, try to appeal to the nurse's professional strengths. Nurses are trained to be patient educators and, when necessary, advocates. If you engage the nurse's role as educator, you can create an ally instead of an adversary.

NURSE: Okay, Mrs. Watson, we're going to send you down to radiology for some X rays. The orderly will be here in a few minutes.

PATIENT: Allison, I'm a little confused here. Could you help me understand something?

NURSE: Sure, Mrs. Watson. What seems to be the problem?

PATIENT: I came in last week for X rays. So why do I need more?

NURSE: Well, it's up to the radiologist. He ordered a set of X rays.

PATIENT: I understand that. But you know a lot about this condition. Do people usually get a second set of X rays a week apart?

NURSE: No, not usually.

PATIENT : And my doctor said I wouldn't need more X rays. Do you think it's possible that the radiologist didn't know I already had X rays taken?

NURSE: I suppose it's possible . . .

PATIENT: Do you think you could check with the radiologist? Because I really don't want to have these X rays if I don't need them. Cancer runs in my family, so I'm concerned about radiation.

NURSE: Let me make a phone call.

This approach won't always work. But you'll stand a better chance of getting what you need if you work to make the nurse your ally instead of your adversary. It's harder for a nurse to turn her back on a patient who needs help than on one who's seen as difficult or uncooperative. You can use this approach with doctors, too. Don't try to tell them how to do their job, or imply that they're uncaring or incompetent. Instead, play the role of student.

Another approach is to use "reflective listening." This technique involves reflecting back what the other person says. It helps ensure that you truly understand what you're hearing. Equally important, it shows that you respect the listener.

Here's an example that uses both the "student" technique and reflective listening.

DOCTOR: I recommend a total knee replacement.

PATIENT: May I ask you a question? I found some information about partial knee replacements. Would that be an option for me?

DOCTOR: I don't recommend them. Once we go in, you're better off replacing the entire knee. You don't want us to have to go back in later.

PATIENT: So from your perspective, it's better to replace the whole knee so I don't need another operation later?

DOCTOR: Exactly.

PATIENT: I understand. But it seems like there are two points of view on this issue. Can you help me understand the other point of view?

DOCTOR: Well, a partial knee replacement is less radical surgery, so recovery time is shorter. And the knee isn't as stiff afterward.

PATIENT: I see. So the tradeoff is faster recovery and better function, but I might have to get the operation redone?

DOCTOR: In a nutshell, yes.

In this exchange, the patient first asks questions to make sure he or she understands what the doctor is saying. Equally important, these questions let the doctor know that the patient understands the options and is prepared to make an informed decision. Even if the patient chooses not to follow the doctor's recommendation, both patient and doctor are working together to arrive at a decision.

4

Know Your Rights

You have the same rights inside a hospital as you do walking down the street.

Knowing that simple fact can go a long way toward making your hospital stay safer. For example, nobody is allowed to touch you without your permission—not to give you an injection, not to check your bandage, not to operate on you. (That doesn't mean a nurse has to ask permission every time she examines you. Your permission is implied if you don't object. But if you refuse permission, nobody can do anything to you.) Nobody can hold you in the hospital against your will. Nobody can force you to accept a treatment you don't want—even if he or she says you need it to save your life.

The hospital will also give you a Patient's Bill of Rights. Read it and understand it. You have the right to be treated with dignity and respect when you're hospitalized. You have the right to know what's being done to you. And (assuming you're a legally competent adult) no one in the hospital can force you to take any drugs, or submit to any tests or procedures, against your will. Say no until you're satisfied that you know what's going on.

The bottom line: You retain power over your body—at least as long as you can make your wishes known. The choices are always yours.

A Patient's Bill of Rights

Most hospitals provide patients with a "bill of rights" based on this model from the American Hospital Association. Keep a copy close by and make sure your health care advocate has one, too. You can use it as a tool to help you get the care you need and deserve.

Effective health care requires collaboration between patients and physicians and other health care professionals. Open and honest communication, respect for personal and professional values, and sensitivity to differences are integral to optimal patient care. As the setting for the provision of health services, hospitals must provide a foundation for understanding and respecting the rights and responsibilities of patients, their families, physicians, and other caregivers. Hospitals must ensure a health care ethic that respects the role of patients in decision making about treatment choices and other aspects of their care. Hospitals must be sensitive to cultural, racial, linguistic, religious, age, gender, and other differences as well as the needs of persons with disabilities.

The American Hospital Association presents a Patient's Bill of Rights with the expectation that it will contribute to more effective patient care and be supported by the hospital on behalf of the institution, its medical staff, employees, and patients. The American Hospital Association encourages health care institutions to tailor this bill of rights to their patient community by translating and/or simplifying the language of this bill of rights as may be necessary to ensure that patients and their families understand their rights and responsibilities.

BILL OF RIGHTS
THE PATIENT CARE PARTNERSHIP: UNDERSTANDING EXPECTATIONS, RIGHTS, AND RESPONSIBILITIES

When you need hospital care, your doctor and the nurses and other professionals at our hospital are committed to working with you and your family to meet your health care needs. Our dedicated doctors and staff serve the community in all its ethnic, religious, and economic diversity. Our goal is for you and your family to have the same care and attention we would want for our families and ourselves.

The sections below explain some of the basics about how you can expect to be treated during your hospital stay. They also cover what we will need from you to care for you better. If you have questions at any time, please ask them. Unasked or unanswered questions can add to the stress of being in the hospital. Your comfort and confidence in your care are very important to us.

WHAT TO EXPECT DURING YOUR HOSPITAL STAY

• *High quality hospital care.* Our first priority is to provide you the care you need, when you need it, with skill, compassion, and respect. Tell your caregivers if you have concerns about your care or if you have pain. You have the right to know the identity of doctors, nurses, and others involved in your care, as well as when they are students, residents, or other trainees.

• *A clean and safe environment.* Our hospital works hard to keep you safe. We use special policies and procedures to avoid mistakes in your care and keep you free from abuse or neglect. If anything unexpected and significant happens during your hospital stay, you will be told what happened and any resulting changes in your care will be discussed with you.

• *Involvement in your care.* You and your doctor often make decisions about your care before you go to the hospital. Other times, especially in emergencies, those decisions are made during your hospital stay. When they take place, making decisions should include:

Discussing your medical condition and information about medically appropriate treatment choices. To make informed decisions with your doctor, you need to understand several things:

The benefits and risks of each treatment.

Whether it is experimental or part of a research study.

What you can reasonably expect from your treatment and any long-term effects it might have on your quality of life.

What you and your family will need to do after you leave the hospital.

The financial consequences of using uncovered services or out-of-network providers.

(Please tell your caregivers if you need more information about treatment choices.)

Discussing your treatment plan. When you enter the hospital, you sign a general consent to treatment. In some cases, such as surgery or experimental treatment, you may be asked to confirm in writing that you understand what is planned and agree to it. This process protects your right to consent to or refuse a treatment. Your doctor will explain the medical consequences of refusing recommended treatment. It also protects your right to decide if you want to participate in a research study.

Getting information from you. Your caregivers need complete and correct information about your health and coverage so that they can make good decisions about your care. That includes:

1. Past illnesses, surgeries, or hospital stays.

2. Past allergic reactions.

3. Any medicines or diet supplements (such as vitamins and herbs) that you are taking.

4. Any network or admission requirements under your health plan.

Understanding your health care goals and values. You may have health care goals and values or spiritual beliefs that are important to your well-being. They will be taken into account as much as possible throughout your hospital stay. Make sure your doctor, your family, and your care team know your wishes.

Understanding who should make decisions when you cannot. If you have signed a health care power of attorney stating who should speak for you if you become unable to make health care decisions for yourself, or a "living will" or "advance directive" that states your wishes about end-of-life care, give copies to your doctor, your family and your care team. If you or your family need help making difficult decisions, counselors, chaplains and others are available to help.

• *Protection of your privacy.* We respect the confidentiality of your relationship with your doctor and other caregivers, and the sensitive information about your health and health care that are part of that relationship. State and federal laws and hospital operating policies protect the privacy of your medical information. You will receive a Notice of Privacy Practices that describes the ways that we use, disclose and safeguard patient information and that explains how you can obtain a copy of information from our records about your care.

• *Help preparing you and your family for when you leave the hospital.* Your doctor works with hospital staff and professionals in your community. You and your family also play an important role. The success of your treatment often depends on your efforts to follow medication, diet and therapy plans. Your family may need to help care for you at home.

You can expect us to help you identify sources of follow-up care and to let you know if our hospital has a financial interest in any referrals. As long as you agree we can share information about your care with them, we will coordinate our activities with your caregivers outside the hospital. You can also expect to receive information and, where possible, training about the self-care you will need when you go home.

• *Help with your bill and filing insurance claims.* Our staff will file claims for you with health care insurers or other programs such as Medicare and Medicaid. They will also help your doctor with needed documentation. Hospital bills and insurance coverage are often confusing. If you have questions about your bill, contact our business office. If you need help understanding your insurance coverage or health plan, start with your insurance company or health benefits manager. If you do not have health coverage, we will try to help you and your family find financial help or make other arrangements. We need your help with collecting needed information and other requirements to obtain coverage or assistance.

While you are here, you will receive more detailed notices about some of the rights you have as a hospital patient and how to exercise them. We are always interested in improving. If you have questions, comments, or concerns, please contact _____.

The collaborative nature of health care requires that patients, or their families/surrogates, participate in their care. The effectiveness of care and patient satisfaction with the course of treatment depend, in part, on the patient fulfilling certain responsibilities. Patients are responsible for providing information about past illnesses, hospitalizations, medications, and other matters related to health status. To participate effectively in decision making, patients must be encouraged to take responsibility for requesting additional information or clarification about their health status or treatment when they do not fully understand information and instructions. Patients are also responsible for ensuring that the health care institution has a copy of their written advance directive if they have one. Patients are responsible for informing their physicians and other caregivers if they anticipate problems in following prescribed treatment.

Patients should also be aware of the hospital's obligation to be reasonably efficient and equitable in providing care to other patients and the community. The hospital's rules and regulations are designed to help the hospital meet this obligation. Patients and their families are responsible for making reasonable accommodations to the needs of the hospital, other patients, medical staff, and hospital employees. Patients are responsible for providing necessary information for insurance claims and for working with the hospital to make payment arrangements, when necessary.

A person's health depends on much more than health care services. Patients are responsible for recognizing the impact of their lifestyle on their personal health.

Conclusion

Hospitals have many functions to perform, including the enhancement of health status, health promotion, and the prevention and treatment of injury and disease; the immediate and ongoing care and rehabilitation of patients; the education of health professionals, patients, and the community; and research. All these activities must be conducted with an overriding concern for the values and dignity of patients.

5

Learn the Lay of the Land

Hospitals are, in many ways, a world unto themselves—with their own rules, their own traditions, their own culture. The better you understand how hospitals work, the more effective you can be in getting the system to work for you.

Who's in Charge?

Many patients assume that their doctor is in charge of their hospital care.

Not so. Your physician is responsible for directing your *medical* care but not necessarily your *hospital* care.

Confused? No wonder. It's only natural to think that your doctor is in charge. But for a variety of reasons—historical, economic, and legal—your hospital and your doctor are largely independent of one another.

Don't be misled by the fact that your physician is on the staff at the hospital you go to. That simply means that he or she has hospital privileges—in other words, he or she can admit patients to the hospital, attend to them while they are there, write orders for the nursing staff, and order tests and procedures. *It doesn't mean that the physician is part of the hospital management.*

Your doctor is like a patron at a restaurant, not the chef: He or she can order from the hospital's menu of services but can't cook the food.

With certain exceptions (such as residents), most of the doctors you see during your stay aren't even employees of the hospital. Even a hospital-based physician, such as a radiologist who practices exclusively in one hospital, is often legally part of an independent medical group that provides its services on a contract basis to the hospital.

Here's Why It Matters

- Your physician doesn't supervise the nursing staff. So if you have a problem with your nursing care, it won't do much good to complain to your physician.
- Your physician doesn't supervise other departments, such as radiology or the medical lab that evaluates your tests. If you need an X ray or blood work, it's up to your physician to order it. But by and large, it's up to the hospital to figure out when you're going to get it, who's going to perform it, and how he or she is going to do it.

- By the same token, the hospital isn't in charge of your medical care—that is, what the doctor orders off the menu. For example, if you're having a bad reaction to your medication and would like the nurses to give you something different, it may not be their fault if they come back four hours later with the same medication. They can't change your medication without a doctor's order. (There are some exceptions to this related to "dispense-as-needed" or PRN orders, which we discuss later.)

So Who Runs the Place?

On paper, a hospital is organized like any business, with a typical pyramid-style organizational structure. At the top of the pyramid is the hospital administrator, general manager, or CEO, who's responsible for the overall operation of the hospital.

(By the way, some hospitals are run as nonprofit and some as for-profit businesses. In the old days, there were considerable philosophical and organizational distinctions between the two. But these days, there's little practical difference.)

Next are a variety of administrative and nonclinical departments, such as the billing office, medical records, housekeeping, and so on. For your purposes, you don't have to worry too much about them. They're not involved in direct patient care, so they're not likely to affect your physical well-being.

On the other side of the chart are the clinical departments. Though the details may vary from hospital to hospital, most are organized along the following lines:

- Diagnostic services are primarily responsible for conducting tests and procedures to find out what's wrong with you. For example, the imaging or radiology department takes X rays, CT scans, MRIs, and so on.
- The surgical department is responsible for your care just before, during, and after an operation. It oversees the operating rooms and recovery rooms, as well as preps you for surgery.
- A variety of specialized services (such as maternity, cardiac programs, and various types of intensive care units).
- The general medical-surgical service oversees most ordinary hospital care, including patients who are in for testing and medical treatments, as well as surgical patients before their operations and after they return from the recovery room.
- The nursing service provides nurses to staff all of these departments.

Be Nice to Your Nurse

The backbone of the hospital is the nursing service.

Nurses are responsible for the nuts-and-bolts nursing care you receive during your stay, of course. But in most cases they're also responsible for the day-to-day operation of each unit. So if, for example, the pharmacy makes a mistake with your medications, it's usually up to the nurses to try to get the problem straightened out.

It pays to be nice to them.

They're your most important ally against injury and disease while you're in the hospital. Your doctor outlines your overall plan of care and writes a variety of orders that your nurses follow. But nurses aren't just order takers. They're professionals who are trained to exercise independent judgment to keep you safe and well.

In some hospitals, nurses have the time and energy to put that training and those ideals into practice. But if the nurses who care for you seem stressed, tired, and angry, it pays to be extra vigilant. These are the hospitals where things tend to go wrong.

Unfortunately, that group includes more and more hospitals these days. Nurses bear the brunt of much of what's wrong with hospitals today. They're often overworked and understaffed.

Some of these problems are the result of the cost-cutting pressures and nursing shortages that most hospitals face. Nursing shortages and budget cuts are huge problems in hospitals. Nursing shortages tend to create a vicious circle: With fewer nurses, more of them are overworked, leading to more burnout and more nurses leaving the profession.

Things are changing from the old days of starched caps and white uniforms, and enlightened doctors and administrators are now doing a much better job of giving hospital nurses the respect, authority, and autonomy they need to do their jobs well. Unfortunately, many nurses still have to deal with physicians who expect them to be seen and not heard, and administrators who see them as little more than names on a shift schedule.

And while we haven't seen any studies on the subject, our experience suggests that there's a strong relationship between nurses' job satisfaction and the quality of care they deliver. Where hospitals hire talented and caring nurses, treat them with respect, and provide them with sufficient time, resources, and authority, patients are likely to get extraordinary care.

Types of Nurses

There are different types of nurses in hospitals. It's important to know the differences because many hospitals are using unqualified personnel in positions where their responsibility exceeds their training.

Nurse assistants are not nurses but should have completed a certified nurse assistant course before they are hired to work in a hospital. Nurse assistants help with meals, bathing, bed care, transfer of patients, vital signs, and other nonnursing tasks. They do *not* give medications, provide treatments, change dressings, start IVs, or make calls to your physician. They should not be used to replace a nurse.

Licensed practical nurses (LPNs) receive formal training at state-accredited schools and must pass a state license requirement examination in order to practice. They provide a wide variety of patient care. Each state has a different nurse practice act that outlines the scope of nursing practice. However, each hospital also has the authority to determine what treatments the nurses may provide under the Nurse Practice

Act. LPNs' duties vary greatly from hospital to hospital.

With some exceptions, LPNs are permitted to administer medications. LPNs are not allowed to administer blood products in most states.

LPNs can provide treatments, change dressings, call your doctor and report your condition, and take orders. They can also provide all personal care. LPNs generally must take additional medication administration courses at the hospital or college after graduation before they can administer any medications on the job.

Are LPNs being used in place of a registered nurse? In some places, yes. Beware. If this is the case, you might want to choose another establishment to enter for your care.

A few years ago, the LPNs' days seemed numbered, as assistants took on a lot of the less-skilled duties and hospitals insisted on registered nurses for the rest. But with current shortages and cost constraints, many hospitals are placing LPNs in positions once reserved for registered nurses.

Registered nurses (RNs) complete a course of study that may be two years (associate degree), three years (nursing diploma—though very few schools are left in this category), or four years (bachelor of science degree). All RNs must pass a state licensing examination. An RN may continue on in education and obtain a master's degree or Ph.D. The RN may choose the advanced degree to focus on management, research, or clinical practice.

The bachelor programs provide training in leadership and management focused on patient care, along with all of the other education requirements for a bachelor's degree. Nursing bachelor programs provide nursing courses to prepare the nurse to manage nursing units, coordinate the care of the patients, and step into nursing leadership positions.

Registered nurses know a tremendous amount about health, disease, medical procedures, drugs, and how hospitals work. So in addition to providing your day-to-day care, they're often your best resource for questions about your care and even about what your doctor has told you.

Nurse specialists, or advanced practice nurses, are RNs with a master's degree and a specialty certification in a particular area (such as family nurse practitioner, certified nurse midwife, certified nurse anesthetist, or clinical specialist). Each state recognizes advanced practice nurses with requirements and rules specific to that specialty. These specialists include:

- Certified nurse-midwives, who manage pregnancies and deliver babies.
- Obstetric nurses, who assist in deliveries and provide care to new mothers.
- Nurse anesthetists, who deliver anesthesia to surgical patients.
- Operating room nurses, who assist surgeons in operations.
- Recovery room nurses, who monitor patients immediately after surgery.
- Critical care nurses, who care for extremely ill patients in intensive care units.
- IV nurses, who specialize in running intravenous lines. (Yes, it seems like a narrow specialty, but as you'll see, IVs are a key source of infections and complications. If the hospital uses a special IV team, that's a good sign.)

- Others include cancer specialists, urology, neurology, medical surgical nurse specialists, pediatric specialists, and more.

TIP

If you're receiving care from a nurse specialist rather than a doctor, don't assume it's second-class care. In many ways nurse practitioners do a better job than physicians. Because their specialties are narrower, they have a depth of knowledge and expertise in their fields. They're often more skilled at patient education—explaining what's happening to you. And nursing tends to take a more holistic view of patients, focusing not only on your physical needs but also your emotional well-being and lifestyle issues. Keep in mind, however, that the nursing specialist is not a substitute for the doctor. They work together in a collaborative relationship and often work as a team on certain patient problems. Patients always have the right to ask for the collaborating physician to see them. And the nurse will always seek the physician's assistance for problems outside the scope of his or her training.

Signs of a Good Nursing Staff

Here are some ways you can tell that nurses are getting the support they need from the hospital.

They're prompt. Some delays are unavoidable in hospitals. If there's an emergency in another patient's room or an unexpected rush of admissions, nurses may have to postpone routine nursing tasks until they get the situation under control. But if nurses are *constantly* running late with medications and other tasks, it probably means they're spread too thin.

They're mostly RNs. Is most of your care provided by RNs, or by LPNs or nursing assistants? Hospitals may try to stretch thin nursing staffs—and save money—by using less qualified help. If the hospital has an all-RN nursing staff, that's an excellent sign of quality.

They go home at the end of the shift. If you notice that a lot of nurses are working double shifts or putting in overtime, it probably means the staff is shorthanded. Nearly every hospital has to deal with nursing shortages these days, but those that take good care of their nurses can attract and keep staff, so they're less likely to have to resort to mandatory overtime and extra shifts to keep their units staffed. Long hours are a key reason why nurses get burned out and why more errors occur.

They're empowered. Good hospitals give nurses enough flexibility to do a good job and don't impose a lot of needless rules and restrictions. For example, we've seen hospitals that allowed only one parent to stay overnight with a sick infant, even when the child was in a private room. Empowered nurses will be able to bend these kinds of rules to accommodate the family's needs.

They communicate. Good nurses give you information and keep you up to date. Nurses who are stressed or worried about their jobs will be more closemouthed.

THE NURSE-PATIENT RATIO DEBATE

California recently passed legislation requiring hospitals to maintain certain minimum staffing levels for nurses. Similar legislation is being considered in many other states as well.

The legislation has prompted considerable debate. Not surprisingly, hospitals were pushing for lower nurse-to-patient ratios (that is, fewer nurses per patient). The nurses' union wanted higher ratios (more nurses per patient). The final legislation ended up in between.

For instance, in the medical-and-surgical, telemetry (where coronary patients are monitored via television screens), and specialty-care units, the union wanted one nurse for every three patients. The California Hospital Association suggested a one-to-ten ratio. The state announced ratios of one-to-six for medical-and-surgical and one-to-five for telemetry and specialty-care units. Operating room patients under anesthesia and trauma patients in the emergency room require a one-to-one ratio. The ratio is set at one-to-two for labor-and-delivery units, postanesthesia, critical-care, burn, and neonatal intensive care units.

While it's probably a good idea to establish a minimum staffing level, nurses in California and elsewhere are concerned that hospitals may consider these ratios as *caps*—in other words, that they won't add any more nurses than the law requires.

A similar program in Australia, however, has apparently worked well, and the improved working conditions are credited with attracting 10 percent of nurses who had left the profession to return to the field.

Who Else Provides Your Care?

You may also encounter these practitioners during your stay.

The hospital pharmacist. Though you're unlikely ever to meet the hospital pharmacist face to face, he or she is one of the people most responsible for your health during your hospital stay. Pharmacists are licensed by the state and have a degree in pharmacy. Often they're even more knowledgeable than the physician about the drugs you're taking. They do more than just put medications in little paper cups. They're responsible for programs to reduce medication errors and avoid drug interactions, they serve as consultants on medication treatments and management of medications, and they serve as part of the patient care team for quality care, as well as helping to educate nurses and other hospital staff about medications.

Therapists, such as respiratory therapists and physical therapists, are neither physicians nor nurses. They have a college degree (and sometimes a graduate degree) in their specialties. In a hospital, you're most likely to encounter a respiratory therapist if you have breathing problems, or a physical therapist to help you recover from problems with joints or muscles (for example, after a hip replacement). Like nurses and physicians, therapists are highly trained and licensed by the state.

Technicians have skilled specialties but may not be licensed by the state. Many technicians complete a course or school of study in the specialty area; examples include laboratory, X ray, ultrasound, radiation therapy. They usually do the "hands-on" work with various types of medical equipment. For example, if you need an X ray, a radiology technician will set up the equipment, position you, and take the X ray. A *radiologist*—a physician—will actually read the X-ray film and make the diagnosis. Except in an emergency, that step usually takes place later, often at the radiologist's office, and you may never meet the radiologist who reads your X ray.

A technician can answer many of your general questions about procedures but probably won't know much about your condition. Because a technician sees lots of patients, one after the other, make sure he or she knows who you are and what procedure you need to have done. If something seems wrong—if you're having problems with your left knee and the technician wants to give you a chest X ray, for example—don't hesitate to insist that he or she double-check. If necessary, you can refuse the procedure until you're sure.

Patient service representative isn't really a clinical position; it's more of a customer-service function. The patient representative is a sort of all-around ombudsman/problem solver, who may be able to help you cut through red tape or provide answers when you feel you're getting the runaround. When you're having trouble getting problems solved through regular channels, ask if the hospital has a patient representative who can talk to you. Representatives' clout in the hospital hierarchy is usually pretty limited, though. They're more effective at solving minor problems—for example, straightening out your billing—than at taking on the medical or nursing staff.

The Big Picture

It's true that most hospitals are bureaucratic and institutional. They have to be. It's the only practical way to orchestrate all of these various roles and functions and deliver them to a constantly changing clientele day in and day out. By understanding who does what, you're more likely to get the answers you need. And you're better able to tell when things aren't right—and when you may be at increased risk.

6

Choose Your Hospital

In an emergency, you may not have time to choose your hospital. But when you do have a choice—for example, when you're going in for elective surgery—it pays to do your homework. Research shows that the quality of hospitals varies greatly, and that it's possible to identify hospitals that consistently provide better care.

What Are Your Choices?

If you've already selected your surgeon or other specialist, your choices will be limited to hospitals where the doctor has privileges (see Chapter 7). Sometimes it's better to work the other way around: Find a hospital that's good at treating your condition, then find a doctor or doctors with privileges there.

But that's only one consideration. It's also important to consider the hospital's overall track record and reputation. Other factors are important to consider as well: For example, is the hospital conveniently located for family and visitors?

Your health plan may restrict your choices. But if you have a choice of plans, you can look for one that has the hospital you prefer in its network.

QUICK CHECK FOR QUALITY

The Agency for Healthcare Research and Quality, a federal agency that aims to improve the quality of health care, recommends that patients look for a hospital that:

- is accredited by the Joint Commission on Accreditation of Healthcare Organizations
- is rated highly by state or consumer or other groups
- is one where your doctor has privileges, if that is important to you
- is covered by your health plan
- has experience with your condition
- has had success in treating your condition
- checks and works to improve its own quality of care

Strategies for Choosing the Best Hospital

Which hospital is "best"? That depends on a lot of things. For example, a hospital may be very good at treating some diseases and only so-so at others. The choice also depends on what's important to *you*. You may want a hospital that's close by, or that's easy for loved ones to get to, or that's affiliated with a medical school, or where you know a nurse on staff who can look out for you. There's no simple answer, but these strategies can help you make the right decision.

Visit the hospital. Some hospitals offer tours to prospective patients, or will arrange one if you ask (check with the hospital information desk). You can also find out a lot (perhaps even more) simply by showing up. Find out when visiting hours are and stop by. If you know which unit you'll be on, visit it; otherwise, just look for the general medical-surgical unit. Is the unit clean and well organized? Are the nurses relaxed and friendly, or sullen and overworked? If you have questions, approach the nursing station and explain that you're scheduled to be admitted soon. Do the nurses answer your questions or ignore you?

Find Out How the Hospital Ranks on National Quality Standards

Virtually every hospital is surveyed by the Joint Commission on Accreditation of Healthcare Organizations (JCAHO). JCAHO accreditation is required to participate in Medicare and in most private insurance plans. Reviews are done at least every three years.

But even though nearly all hospitals are accredited, not all of them meet the same quality standards. JCAHO has several levels of accreditation, based on how well the hospital performs in a variety of areas. The standards address the quality of staff and equipment, and—most recently—the hospital's success in treating and curing.

JCAHO prepares a performance report on each hospital that it surveys. The report lists

- accreditation status (six levels, from the lowest, "Not Accredited," to the highest, "Accredited with Commendation")
- date of the survey
- evaluation of the key areas reviewed during the survey
- results of any follow-up activity
- areas needing improvement
- comparison with national results

These reports give you a detailed look at how well the hospital performs and a good way to compare one hospital against another. You can order JCAHO's performance reports free by calling 630-792-5800. Or check JCAHO's Web site at http://www.jcaho.org for a hospital's performance report and its accreditation status. (Also see the Resources section on page 222.)

Find Out How Well the Hospital Controls Infections

Infections are one of the biggest risks in hospitals (see Chapter 11), and some hospitals are better than others at controlling them. Hospitals keep track of their infection rates, but these statistics are hard to find. And they would be misleading, anyway, since they're affected in part by the patient mix. Hospitals that care for sicker and older patients tend to have higher rates, no matter how good they are at fighting infection.

The JCAHO ratings, however, are a good way to judge hospitals' efforts at fighting infection. JCAHO doesn't publish hospitals' individual infection rates; instead, it assigns the hospital an infection-control score based on overall efforts at fighting infection.

Check on the Hospital-Nurse Relationship

Because nurses are so critical to hospitals, it's useful to know the state of the relationship between the nursing staff and the hospital administration. Neither the hospital nor nurses are likely to come out and tell you if you ask, but it may be worth doing some digging. For example, if you know any nurses at other local hospitals, ask them about your hospital's reputation among nurses in the area. The grapevine among nurses is usually pretty strong.

You can also research your local newspaper to see if there have been any recent strikes or labor disputes at the hospital (most newspapers allow you to search their back issues on the Web). And, of course, you can ask your doctor about the quality and morale of the nursing staff. Ask him or her which local hospitals have the best nursing staff.

Best Nursing Staffs

The American Nurses Association maintains a list of "magnet centers" that are recognized for providing high-quality nursing care. (You can find more details at http://www.ana.org/ancc/magnet/magnet2.htm.)

Ask How the Nursing Service Is Organized

Hospitals use one of two basic approaches to organizing their nursing staffs: the team nursing and primary nursing models. If you can choose a hospital, look for one where the nursing service is organized on a primary nursing model.

Team nursing is the more traditional approach. All of the nurses in a unit care for their patients as a team. So, you may receive your medications from one nurse on Tuesday morning and from another on Wednesday morning, depending on who's available at the time. The advantage of the team approach is flexibility: Any nurse can be assigned as needed to handle the tasks at hand. As a result, this model tends to be less costly to hospitals, so you don't need as many nurses per patient.

In the primary nursing model, an individual nurse is assigned as the lead during your hospital stay, with an associate for when the primary nurse is off duty. Nurses still work as a team, but your primary nurse manages your entire hospital stay. And because the primary nurse is more familiar with your case, there's less chance of miscommunication and mistakes.

Most nurses feel that primary nursing is a better way

to care for patients. Over the years, more and more hospitals adopted it. But now many of them have switched back to team nursing because of cost and the difficulty of recruiting nurses.

If you're in a hospital that uses this model, find out who your primary nurse will be and provide any information that will help him or her manage your care—for example, your medical history and your questions and concerns. Don't assume that your primary nurse understands all of these details, no matter how many people you've told already or whether it's already in your chart. Primary nurses are busy and overworked, too, and it's important for them to see the big picture—from your perspective.

Find Out How the Hospital Compares with Others in Your Area

Hospital "report cards" are available from a number of sources. Pennsylvania, California, and Ohio have laws that require hospitals to report data on the quality of their care. You can get this information from your state's health department or, often, from the hospitals themselves.

Some local consumer groups also gather information on how well hospitals perform and how satisfied their patients are. One example is the Cleveland Health Quality Choice Program, which is made up of businesses, doctors, and hospitals. Consumer groups publish guides to hospitals and other health care choices in various cities. Find out what kind of information is available where you live by calling your state department of health, health care council, or hospital association.

U.S. News & World Report publishes an annual "Best Hospitals" guide, ranking 205 hospitals in 17 specialties. (That's just a small fraction of the 6,000-plus hospitals in the United States.) The report uses a ranking system that considers the hospital's reputation (as reported by physicians), mortality (the number of deaths, adjusted for the type of patients that the hospital serves), and other factors from the American Hospital Association's annual survey of hospitals. You can find the rankings on-line at www.usnews.com.

Also, ask your doctor what he or she thinks about the hospitals you're considering. Your doctor may not want to say a particular hospital is good or bad. Instead, ask which hospital he or she prefers, and why.

Find Out Whether the Hospital Has Experience with Your Condition

General hospitals handle a wide range of routine conditions, such as hernias and pneumonia. Specialty hospitals have a lot of experience with certain conditions (such as cancer) or certain groups (such as children). General hospitals may also have specialized units or programs.

Also find out the level of the hospital. Smaller community hospitals may not be well equipped to handle certain diseases or conditions. Or they may not have the resources to treat you if complications develop or your condition worsens, meaning you'd have to be transferred to another hospital. Tertiary care hospitals offer the highest level of care.

Research shows that hospitals that do many of the same types of procedures tend to have better success with them. Practice makes perfect. Ask your doctor or the hospital if there is information on:

- how often the procedure is done there
- how often the doctor and support team (for example, the surgical team) perform the procedure
- the patient outcomes (how well the patients do)

Some state and local health departments publish reports on *outcomes studies* for specific procedures. These studies show, for example, how well patients at a given hospital do after having heart bypass surgery. Such studies can help you compare which hospitals and surgeons have had the most success with a procedure.

Getting a Hospital Report Card from JCAHO

To get a performance report on a hospital from the Joint Commission on Accreditation of Healthcare Organizations, start by going to the JCAHO Web site at www.jcaho.org.

At the Web site, click on the Quality Check button under Accredited Organizations. That will take you to a search screen.

You can search for hospitals in several ways. To find all of the hospitals in your county, for example, enter your state in the Geographic Location box and your county in the County box. Make sure the form says Hospitals in the Type of Organization box. Then click on the Search button.

You'll get a list of hospitals. Click on the name of any hospital and you'll be sent to a summary page for the hospital. (Warning: To search multiple hospitals, you need to start over each time. The Back button on your browser won't work.)

The summary page will tell you the hospital's current accreditation status. Here are definitions of the terms.

Accreditation with Commendation used to be the highest level of accreditation, for hospitals that demonstrated "more than satisfactory compliance" with applicable Joint Commission standards in all performance areas on a complete accreditation survey before January 1, 2000. Although this decision category has been discontinued, hospitals that earned this designation get to keep it until their next survey unless performance slips in the meantime.

Accreditation with Full Standards Compliance is the highest level awarded. The hospital demonstrates satisfactory compliance with applicable Joint Commission standards in all performance areas.

Accreditation with Requirements for Improvement (formerly Accreditation with Type I Recommendations) is awarded to hospitals that demonstrate satisfactory compliance with applicable Joint Commission standards in most performance areas but have deficiencies in one or more performance areas or in meeting accreditation policy requirements. The deficiencies must be resolved within a specified time period.

Each year, 5 percent of all organizations are selected for random, unannounced surveys of standards for known problem areas. These surveys take place nine to thirty months following the three-year full survey. In addition, the Joint

Commission conducts for-cause unannounced surveys in response to serious incidents relating to the health and/or safety of patients or staff, or reported complaints. The outcomes of these surveys may affect the current accreditation status of an organization.

Accreditation Watch. Though not a separate accreditation decision, JCAHO will place an organization on accreditation watch when it has not completed a timely, thorough, and credible analysis and action plan for any sentinel event occurring there (sentinel events are specific high-risk events that the commission monitors).

Preliminary Denial of Accreditation occurs rarely, when JCAHO concludes that the hospital hasn't complied with standards in multiple performance areas or accreditation policy requirements, or for other reasons. This accreditation decision is subject to subsequent review.

Provisional Accreditation is for new or previously unaccredited hospitals that show satisfactory compliance during a preliminary on-site evaluation. It remains in effect until a complete survey is performed.

Areas Having Specific Recommendations for Improvement is a list of the performance areas in which recommendations for improvement have been identified. A recommendation for improvement is provided when a health care organization does not demonstrate adequate compliance with specific Joint Commission standards. An accredited organization must resolve recommendations for improvement within a specified period of time to remain accredited. As an organization improves its performance in an area, "RESOLVED" is displayed to the right of the performance area on the performance report.

Overall Evaluation Score

The report also lists an overall score for the organization. It is based on a scale of 0 to 100, with 100 representing the highest possible score. Nearly two-thirds of all hospitals score 90 or above.

The smaller the differences in scores among organizations, the less likely there is an actual difference in their levels of performance. There may be no real difference between an organization that scores 88 and an organization that scores 81. However, the greater the difference in scores, the more likely there is a difference in patient care.

The Joint Commission doesn't grade on a curve. That is, the scoring doesn't indicate an organization's ranking in relation to others. Rather, the score indicates how well it measures up against an absolute "perfect" standard.

Updated Overall Evaluation Score

The Updated Overall Evaluation Score provided on performance reports is calculated after follow-up and other monitoring assessments have been conducted. The updated score assumes continued standards compliance in those performance areas which were in compliance at the time of the original full survey. The maximum score that can be achieved is 94.

Some organizations demonstrate acceptable (significant) but not total compliance at the time of their full surveys, and they are not assigned follow-up activities. In these instances, an Updated Overall Evaluation Score is usually not provided.

Some organizations achieve an overall evaluation score greater than or equal to 94 at the time of their full surveys. If they are assigned follow-up activities, individual performance area scores are updated to reflect improvement, but an updated overall score is not provided because the original score equals or exceeds 94.

Digging Deeper

For more details on the hospital, look on the left of the hospital's page, under "Contents." Find the section that says, "The following performance reports are available for this organization." Under this heading, "Hospital services" gives you an overall report, with details on each "performance area" in the hospital.

Here's how to interpret the report.

Performance Area Scores. Each performance area in the hospital is scored at the time of the full survey. This score is indicated in the "Full Survey Performance Area Scores" column. Scores are based on a scale of 1 to 5, with 1 representing the highest possible score. If the score for a specific performance area has been updated, this updated score appears in the "Updated Performance Area Scores" column.

Definitions of the scores:

Score 1—Substantial compliance. The organization consistently meets all major provisions of the standards in this performance area.

Score 2—Significant compliance. The organization meets most provisions of the standards in this performance area.

Score 3—Partial compliance. The organization meets some provisions of the standards in this performance area.

Score 4—Minimal compliance. The organization meets few provisions of the standards in this performance area.

Score 5—Noncompliance. The organization fails to meet the provisions of the standards in this performance area.

NA—Not applicable. The performance area does not apply to the organization.

Updated Performance Scores. This column on a performance report shows the most recent performance of the health care organization and includes updates that have occurred since the full survey.

7

Choose Your Physicians

One of the greatest risks during a hospital stay is uncoordinated care—basically, the left hand not knowing what the right hand is doing. Various doctors and therapists troop in and out, each focused on his or her narrow specialty. But nobody is putting all the pieces into a comprehensive plan of care that reflects what you need and want.

The best way to avoid these problems is by having a physician who knows you and your medical needs. Patients who come into the hospital without a physician are assigned, more or less at random, to an attending physician on the hospital staff. The attending may be a terrific doctor, but he or she doesn't know about your background or medical history beyond what's in your chart. He or she may have a practice style that isn't in line with your expectations. And his or her focus is limited to what happens to you while you're in the hospital, not your ongoing needs.

In short, it's better to choose your doctor than have one chosen for you.

Primary-Care Physicians, Attendings, and Specialists

There are three categories of physicians who should be involved in your hospital care:

Your *primary-care* physician is your regular doctor, the one you go to for checkups and routine health care, and who treats you year in and year out. He or she is primary in the sense of being your first stop in the health care system and ultimately responsible for coordinating all of your care. Primary-care physicians are often family practice physicians, but they may be any type of specialist. If you have a chronic heart condition, for example, your cardiologist may act as your primary-care physician. HMOs and other managed-care plans often require you to choose a primary-care physician who acts as a gatekeeper, determining which kind of specialty care you need and arranging for any referrals.

Your *attending* physician is the doctor who's in charge of your hospital stay. It may or may not be your primary-care physician, depending on where you go and what you're being treated for. Often, this will be a specialist who's been treating you already—for example, a cardiologist for heart problems, or an oncologist for cancer.

Your hospital may offer a relatively new option for an attending physician, especially if you need intensive care: a *hospitalist.*

Hospitalists are physicians who work only in the hospital. When you're admitted to the ICU, your attending physician turns your care over to the hospitalist. Hospitalists staff the units they work in twenty-four hours a day and are readily available to examine you and manage your care. The nurses don't need to wait for a return call from your attending physician to take care of a problem.

If you're transferred from the ICU to a medical or surgical unit, a hospitalist may continue to manage your hospital stay. After discharge, your primary physician resumes your care. This approach benefits you. Outcomes of critical illness improve because of the consistency of care and the level of expertise of the hospitalist.

Finally, there are other *specialists* who may be involved in your care, physicians with special expertise in a particular area. For surgery, you will have an anesthesiologist. If you have X rays, a radiologist will read them and report on his or her findings. If you have a biopsy taken, a pathologist will study the tissue and make a report as well. Your attending physician may also seek consultations from other specialists with special expertise. You may never meet some of these specialists. Others may stop by your room once or twice, or order some additional tests. They're all part of your team. If you have any questions about them—who they are, what their role is, or what they've recommended—ask your attending physician.

Choosing Your Primary-Care Physician

Start by choosing your primary-care physician, if you haven't already. You should have a primary health care provider even if you're healthy. By establishing a relationship with a health care provider, you get to know the medical personnel and how the system works. Your insurance company may require you to choose a primary-care physician from an approved list. You can choose a doctor who's not on the list, of course, but the insurance company may not pay for his or her services (or may pay at a reduced rate).

Your primary-care physician is the linchpin in the system, so it's important to find one with whom you see eye to eye. Even if your health plan doesn't require you to choose a primary-care doctor, it's a good idea to select one. Studies show that people who have a regular doctor get better care and are likely to stay healthier than people who look for a doctor only when they're sick.

Choosing a Specialist

Your primary-care physician, in turn, will help you select the team that will treat you in the hospital—including an attending physician if necessary, any specialists you may need, anesthesiologists, and so forth.

You can and should be an active partner with your primary-care physician in assembling the team. Don't be shy about asking your primary-care physician tough questions about the specialists he or she recommends. Ultimately, the decision is yours. You may be limited to who's in your insurer's network and by who has privileges at the hospital you go to, but you should have a number of choices. If you need a treatment or procedure that's not widely available, talk to your doctor and insurance company; in those circumstances insurers sometimes pay to send you to an out-of-network hospital or specialist.

When choosing a specialist, you can do some independent research to find the doctor you want.

You can ask friends, colleagues, or coworkers for recommendations. Remember that these opinions are based on personal experiences, and not everyone has an objective opinion. Ask nurses who work in the hospital; they're medically knowledgeable and work closely with physicians. Their views are usually unbiased—they have nothing to gain or lose by giving you an honest opinion—and they are usually well informed. Rather than asking them whether a certain doctor is good or bad, simply ask which doctor they'd choose if they needed a specialist.

Your local medical society has a list of doctors in the area and their specialties, where they practice, and how to get in touch with them. But it won't make recommendations one way or the other.

You can check to see if anyone has rated doctors in your area, such as a consumer group or a local magazine. Information on doctors in certain states is available at www.docboard.com, a Web site run by a group of state medical board directors. Another source is a series of "best doctor" guides from Castle Connolly Medical Ltd. It publishes *America's Top Doctors: The Best in American Medicine,* as well as several regional guides. They're available at bookstores or amazon.com.

You can also ask about the practice that the physician belongs to. A large multispecialty group practice, for example, gives you a "one-stop shop" if you need other specialists. On the other hand, a small practice or solo practitioner may give you more personalized care. Find out who covers for your doctor when he or she is unavailable. Nonmedical factors may come into play as well: Is the doctor so busy that it's hard to get an appointment? (If so, your treatment may be delayed.) Is the staff knowledgeable and helpful?

In some states, you can check if lawsuits have been filed against a doctor. This information is in the public domain, but it's usually not worth researching, because it's often misleading. A doctor may be sued even though he or she did nothing wrong. Malpractice lawyers often name as many defendants as possible—even doctors who were only marginally involved in the case—to create "deeper pockets" for a judgment or settlement and, sometimes, as a tactic to gather information or pressure doctors to testify against their colleagues. An insurance company may settle a case even when wrongdoing is doubtful, simply to avoid the costs of an expensive court battle. And if a doctor has a clean malpractice record, it may simply mean he or she hasn't been practicing as long!

Choosing a Surgeon

Surgery is as much art as science. Surgeons must know not only what to do; they must also have the ability to perform the procedure flawlessly. Like an athlete's, a surgeon's talent is part a physical skill and part a mental one. Surgeons must, of course, have good technical knowledge. But they must also have sure hands and the ability to make good decisions quickly and under pressure.

With athletes, it's easy to tell who's the best. You just look at the statistics. But there are no equivalent stats that you can compare for surgeons. No central clearinghouse tracks how many operations a surgeon has performed, or how successful those operations were. And anyway, comparisons would be virtually meaningless because so many other factors are involved: How old were the patients? Were they in relatively good health to begin with? Which hospitals did patients recover in? You might find, in fact, that the best surgeons have lower success rates—because they get the toughest cases. So you have to use other ways to tell whether you're getting a good surgeon.

Start by getting as much information as you can from your regular doctor. For elective surgery, your regular doctor will probably give you a referral. Ask for more than one recommendation, if possible.

Also ask your doctor for a frank assessment of the surgeon: Why did he or she recommend this surgeon? Is it simply because it's the one your health plan wants you to use? Has your doctor sent other patients there? For similar conditions? Does your doctor know the surgeon's track record?

Ask whether your surgeon is board certified in surgery. A board-certified physician receives specialized training and must undergo periodic examinations to ensure that his or her knowledge is up-to-date. The American Board of

Medical Specialties (800-733-2267) can tell you whether a physician is board certified, and in what specialty. Some surgeons also have the letters F.A.C.S. after their name. This means they are Fellows of the American College of Surgeons and have passed another review by surgeons of their surgical practices.

When you meet the surgeon, try to get a sense of his or her approach. Does he or she *listen?* Does he or she respect your concerns and your wishes, or brush aside your questions with an I'm-the-expert attitude? It's important for the surgeon to understand what you want. You, not the surgeon, are the one who has to live with the results.

Is the surgeon straightforward and open? The surgeon shouldn't hesitate to give you information—good or bad. Think twice about a surgeon who simply tells you not to worry.

Practice makes perfect among surgeons. Studies show that error rates go way down when surgeons and hospitals do a given operation frequently. Ask how often the surgeon and the surgical team have performed the procedure you're about to undergo. Also ask how recent this experience is (the more recent, the better).

Finally, ask who will actually perform the surgery. Will it be the surgeon you meet? Someone else in the practice? A resident under the surgeon's direction? In many hospitals a surgical resident—a licensed physician who's training to become a surgeon—may perform all or part of the operation under your surgeon's supervision. That's how doctors learn to do surgery. But it means that after all your work to select a surgeon, you may actually be getting someone with far less experience. For elective surgery, you have the right to insist on who will do the operation. Make sure it's spelled out in writing on the consent forms you sign—and make a point of telling the surgeon.

COVERING UP INCOMPETENCE

One place not to ask when you're choosing a doctor is the hospital or clinic where he or she practices. It won't tell you whether there have been problems with a physician. Hospitals, clinics, and physicians go to great lengths to protect themselves. Even if everyone knows about a problem, little may be done to remove or discipline the doctor.

I once worked with a physician I'll call Dr. X. He admitted patients to the intensive care unit (ICU) and often wrote inappropriate orders for patients. Nurses repeatedly had to go over his head and talk to the director of the department to protect their patients from bad medical decisions.

Dr. X's medical mistakes caused complications and prolonged patients' hospital stays, yet he was never disciplined or had his privileges revoked. After repeated incidents, the hospital tried to cover itself—but quietly. Dr. X wasn't disciplined or dismissed from the hospital staff, although he wasn't allowed to admit patients to the ICU unless another attending physician gave orders for the patient.

Dr. X was strange in other ways, too. He frequently asked nurses bizarre, paranoid questions that had nothing to do with patient care. For example, when housekeepers used vacuum cleaners, Dr. X insisted that they were part of a plot to get him and "steal all my secrets." He actually reported the housekeepers to the hospital administration.

I was the house supervisor one Saturday morning when Dr. X made rounds. Shortly after he appeared on the floor, two nurses paged me in a panic. Dr. X had threatened to kill them when they left the hospital because he didn't like the way they'd been looking at him! Enraged and fearful for the safety of staff and patients, I immediately called security to look for Dr. X. I had a guard posted in the nursing unit until we'd established that Dr. X had left the building. Then I called all the administrators of the hospital and the medical staff director, and told the of the incident. I had the nurses document the incident and made copies. Witnesses gave written statements as well.

Within a few hours, Dr. X's hospital privileges were revoked, his patients were assigned to other physicians, and he was forced to seek psychiatric counseling. All's well that ends well, I suppose—but everybody knew that Dr. X had been a ticking time bomb and nothing had been done.

His hospital privileges were never reinstated and his practice soon closed. *But his license to practice medicine was never revoked.* He could well be practicing medicine somewhere else today.

What to Tell the Doctors Before You're Admitted

The more information you share with your doctors before you go into the hospital, the better job they can do. Tell as much as you know. You may have to cover the same ground several times for the different specialists as well as nurses; don't assume that they'll share information.

Include any hospitalizations, operations (done in or out of the hospital), and injuries or illnesses you've had. Bring old medical records and test results if you have them. Tell the doctor about any other care you're now receiving and who's providing it—not just physicians, but also chiropractors, herbalists, and so on.

Tell the doctor about your current and past medications. Bring a list of medications you're now taking (including vitamins and over-the-counter and herbal/natural remedies), including how much you take and how often. Tell him or her about any allergies of which you're aware. If you smoke, drink alcohol, use recreational drugs, or are at risk for HIV, tell the doctor. Any information you provide to your doctor is confidential, and you're putting your health at risk if your doctor doesn't know.

Ask Questions!

For a variety of reasons, many patients are reluctant to ask the doctor any questions: They're worried that the doctor will get angry at being second-guessed or that they're bothering the doctor. Some patients don't want to seem ignorant. Or they are afraid of an answer they don't want to hear. Sometimes the doctor seems intimidating. Patients frequently ask the nurse their questions instead of the physician. We provide what answers we are able to and suggest that the patient write down any questions they want to ask the doctor.

If there's one thing you can do to improve your health care, it's to ask your doctor questions. The doctor is working for *you*. You're entitled to information about your body.

When you're choosing a doctor, you can ask anything that comes to mind. Here are some key questions:

- What's wrong with me? (Amazingly, many patients never ask this question.)
- How will you treat it?
- What drugs will you prescribe? How will they help me? What are their side effects?
- What are the treatments going to be and what are the side effects and outcomes of treatments?
- How long will I have to stay in the hospital?
- Will I need to go to another hospital for special care?

Bring a notepad and take notes. Or use a tape recorder. If you've chosen a health care advocate, ask him or her to come with you so he or she will know what's supposed to happen to you in the hospital.

If necessary, ask for written instructions. If you want additional information, ask the doctor where you can get it. For example, does the doctor keep a list of self-help or patient organizations for people with your condition? Is the doctor involved with these groups? Nurses can also give you information about these groups.

8

Make Sure Your Wishes Will Be Followed

Hospitals seem to require an endless stream of paperwork.

We won't go into all of the countless forms you'll be asked to fill out and sign when you go into the hospital. But two items—your medical power of attorney and your living will—can be critical to your well-being when you're in the hospital.

It's best to take care of these documents before you go into the hospital—or as soon as you can after you're admitted. If something happens to you and you're not able to make decisions about your care, these documents will be enormously important.

Together, these documents help ensure that your wishes about your medical care are respected even if you're unconscious or otherwise unable to say what you want. The *living will* spells out these instructions. The *medical power of attorney* appoints someone to make legally binding decisions about your medical care if you become incapacitated.

The Living Will

A living will (also called a healthcare directive or directive to physicians) explains your preferences about certain kinds of medical treatment and life-sustaining procedures if you can't communicate your wishes. If your living will is prepared properly, your doctors are legally bound to respect your wishes or to transfer you to a doctor who will.

Often, living wills are used to instruct doctors to withhold life-prolonging treatments. But some people want to make sure that they get all medical treatment that's available. A living will can do that, too. It's a way to make your wishes known. The living will should be as specific as possible. Bear in mind that your doctor and family will be bound to follow its instructions. Consider, for example, which if any of the following treatments you wish to have if you're terminally ill or comatose:

- blood and blood products
- cardiopulmonary resuscitation (CPR)
- diagnostic tests
- dialysis
- drugs
- respirators
- surgery

Even if you don't want these or other treatments, the laws of most states provide that supportive care, such as food, water, and pain relief, continue to be provided. Some people, however, don't want to have food or fluids if they become comatose or terminally ill, since these procedures may prolong death. You can direct that all food, water, and pain relief be withheld, even if your doctor thinks they're necessary.

Your living will takes effect only when three things occur:

- You're diagnosed to be terminally ill and close to death, or diagnosed to be permanently comatose.
- You can't communicate your wishes about your medical care.
- Your doctor and other medical personnel who are caring for you are informed of the instructions in the living will.

You can insist that your living will be included as part of your medical record when you're admitted. But sometimes these instructions are overlooked or ignored. Just to be sure, it's a good idea to give copies of both your living will and medical power of attorney to family members, the person you designate as your power of attorney, your physician, and any medical clinic and hospital in your area. Be sure to take a copy on vacation. Also, keep one or more copies in your home (not in a safety-deposit box), in a place that you can quickly explain to family members or paramedics in an emergency.

The Medical Power of Attorney

Under the law, there are two types of powers of attorney. A *general* power of attorney gives someone the right to make any legally binding decision on your behalf. A *limited* power of attorney grants someone the authority to make decisions only about certain things.

A medical power of attorney is one type of limited power of attorney. It grants the person you name the legal right to make decisions about your health care—for example, to give permission for you to have an operation. (It *doesn't* give this person control over your finances, access to your checking account, or anything else.)

Unlike a living will, the power of attorney doesn't have to spell out what type of treatment you want or do not want to receive. You can leave those decisions up to the judgment of the person you appoint. Often, however, a living will and medical power of attorney go hand in hand.

The medical power of attorney should explicitly state that it is a *durable* power of attorney, which stays valid even if you become unable to handle your own affairs. If you don't specify that you want your power of attorney to be durable, it will automatically end if you later become incapacitated. (Usually a standard form is used to cover this and other details.)

First, you must choose whom you will name in your medical power of attorney. This person doesn't need to *be* an attorney; in this context it simply means someone empowered to act on your behalf. Nor does the person have to be medically knowledgeable. Most important is whether the person is able to ask the right questions, grasp complex information, carry out your wishes, make good decisions under pressure, and be assertive if necessary.

Often it will be a close family member or next of kin—but it doesn't have to be. Of course, the person you select will likely consult with your other loved ones, but he or she will have the final say about what happens to you. Make sure the person you choose understands this role and is willing to accept it. (Never name someone without discussing it with him or her first.)

The person you select as your health care advocate may also be a good choice to hold power of attorney, but they don't have to be the same person. For example, you might choose a friend who's a nurse to serve as your advocate, because he or she can "talk the talk" and knows how to get things done in the hospital, and someone else, such as a family member, for your medical power of attorney.

If you don't prepare a medical power of attorney, your next of kin will likely be the one to make these decisions on your behalf. In some cases, however—for example, if there's a dispute between your doctors and the family—the whole thing could end up in the courts (these cases are the exception, however). Also, if your partner is not a legal spouse, he or she might not be able to make important decisions for you without a medical power of attorney. Even if you don't prepare a power of attorney, you should still create a living will, to ensure that you get the medical care that you want.

Give the person you name in your power of attorney the tools to do the job. Provide him or her with your doctors' names and phone numbers, including your primary-care physician. Explain your medical history as

much as you can and your understanding of why you're
going into the hospital and what you expect to happen
there.

Above all, explain your wishes. Even though they're
spelled out in your living will, explain them in person, face to
face, and be sure the person understands them. Be specific.
For example, under what circumstances would you want life
support measures to be discontinued? These can be difficult
and emotional discussions, but you don't have to do them
alone. Before you go into the hospital, make an appointment
with your doctor and bring along the person who has your
medical power of attorney to discuss your options. Or if
you're already in the hospital, discuss these issues with the
person you designate and with your doctor and nurse.

Where to Get—and Keep—the Forms

Hospitals and most doctors' offices have fill-in-the-blank
forms to use for creating your medical power of attorney
and living will. You can also get them, and help filling them
out, from your attorney, some senior centers, or other
organizations. The requirements vary slightly from one
state to another, so it's important to use the right forms. To
prove that you were competent to sign the documents, they
must be signed in the presence of witnesses or a notary
public—sometimes both, depending on your state's law. If
you're physically unable to sign but are still able to make
your wishes known verbally, you can have someone else
sign for you—in the presence of witnesses or a notary.

Here is a sample medical power of attorney and living will from the American Medical Association and American Association of Retired Persons (AARP). Most states have specific laws about living wills, and these laws include specific language that should be included in the form. The state forms follow this model pretty closely, but it's best to get a form that's specific for your state. Laws vary from state to state, particularly about the formalities for completion such as witnesses and notaries. For example, California, Ohio, Texas, and Vermont require the use of their state statutory forms, and Michigan requires the agent's signature on the advance directive. Therefore, it is important to seek advice about your own state's law and how it applies to your situation.

You can obtain up-to-date state-by-state information about advance directives, along with statutory forms, if they exist in your state, from:

Legal Counsel for the Elderly (LCE)
American Association of Retired Persons
P.O. Box 96474
Washington, DC 20090–6474

LCE has state-specific guidebooks about advance directives. You can order a booklet for $5 (for shipping and handling) from the above address. Hospital associations, medical societies, or bar associations in your state or county, or your local Area Agency on Aging, or AAA, may provide forms for your state.

If your state has a statutory form, remember that preprinted forms—including the one that's shown here—may not meet all your needs.

Health Care Advance Directive ("Living Will"): Form and Instructions

CAUTION: This health care advance directive is a general form provided for your convenience. Although it meets the legal requirements of most states, it may or may not fit the requirements of your particular state. Many states have special forms or special procedures for creating health care advance directives. Even if your state's law does not clearly recognize this document, it may still provide an effective statement of your wishes if you cannot speak for yourself.

Section 1—Health Care Agent

Print your full name here as the principal or creator of the health care advance directive. Print the full name, address, and telephone number of the person (age eighteen or older) you appoint as your health care agent. Appoint only a person with whom you have talked and whom you trust to understand and carry out your values and wishes.

Many states limit the persons who can serve as your agent. If you want to meet all existing state restrictions, do not name any of the following as your agent, since some states will not let them act in that role:

- your health care providers, including physicians
- staff of health care facilities or nursing care facilities providing your care
- guardians of your finances (also called conservators)
- employees of government agencies financially responsible for your care
- any person serving as agent for ten or more persons

Section 2—Alternate Agents

It is a good idea to name alternate agents in case your first agent is not available. Of course, appoint alternates only if you fully trust them to act faithfully as your agent and you have talked to them about serving as your agent. Print the appropriate information in this paragraph. You can name as many alternate agents as you wish, but place them in the order you wish them to serve.

Section 3—Effective Date and Durability

This sample document is effective if and when you cannot make health care decisions. Your agent and your doctor determine if you are in this condition. Some state laws include specific procedures for determining your decision-making ability. If you wish, you can include other effective dates or other criteria for determining that you cannot make health care decisions (such as requiring two physicians to evaluate your decision-making ability). You also can state that the power will end at some later date or event before death.

In any case, you have the right to revoke or take away the

agent's authority at any time. To revoke, notify your agent or health care provider orally or in writing. If you revoke, it is best to notify in writing both your agent and physician and anyone else who has a copy of the directive. Also destroy the health care advance directive document itself.

Health Care Advance Directive
Part I
Appointment of Health Care Agent

1. HEALTH CARE AGENT

I, _____, hereby appoint:

      PRINCIPAL

_____

      AGENT'S NAME

_____

      ADDRESS

_____

  HOME PHONE #   WORK PHONE #

as my agent to make health and personal care decisions for me as authorized in this document.

2. ALTERNATE AGENTS

IF
—I revoke my Agent's authority; or

—my Agent becomes unwilling or unavailable to act; or

—my Agent is my spouse and I become legally separated
   or divorced

I name the following (each to act alone and successively,
in the order named) as alternates to my Agent:

A. First Alternate Agent _____

Address _____

Telephone _____

B. Second Alternate Agent _____

Address _____

Telephone _____

3. EFFECTIVE DATE AND DURABILITY

By this document I intend to create a health care
advance directive. It is effective upon, and only during,

any period in which I cannot make or communicate a choice regarding a particular health care decision. My Agent, attending physician, and any other necessary experts should determine that I am unable to make choices about health care.

Section 4—Agent's Powers

This grant of power is intended to be as broad as possible. Unless you set limits, your agent will have authority to make any decision you could make to obtain or stop any type of health care.

Even under this broad grant of authority, your agent still must follow your wishes and directions, communicated by you in any manner now or in the future.

To specifically limit or direct your agent's power, you must complete Section 6 in Part II of the advance directive.

---

4. AGENT'S POWERS

I give my Agent full authority to make health care decisions for me. My Agent shall follow my wishes as known to my Agent either through this document or through other means. When my Agent interprets my wishes, I intend my Agent's authority to be as broad as possible, except for any limitations I state in this form. In making any decision, my Agent shall try to discuss the proposed decision with me to determine my desires if I am able to communicate in any way. If my Agent cannot determine the choice I would want, then my Agent shall make a choice for me based upon what my Agent believes to be in my best interests.

Unless specifically limited by Section 6, below, my Agent is authorized as follows:

A.   To consent, refuse, or withdraw consent to any and all types of health care. Health care means any care, treatment, service, or procedure to maintain, diagnose, or otherwise affect an individual's physical or mental condition. It includes, but is not limited to, artificial respiration, nutritional support and hydration, medication, and cardiopulmonary resuscitation;

B.   To have access to medical records and information to the same extent that I am entitled, including the right to disclose the contents to others as appropriate for my health care;

C.   To authorize my admission to or discharge (even against medical advice) from any hospital, nursing home, residential care, assisted living, or similar facility or service;

D.   To contract on my behalf for any health care related service or facility on my behalf, without my Agent incurring personal financial liability for such contracts;

E. To hire and fire medical, social service, and other support personnel responsible for my care;

F. To authorize, or refuse to authorize, any medication or procedure intended to relieve pain, even though such use may lead to physical damage, addiction, or hasten the moment of (but not intentionally cause) my death;

G. To make anatomical gifts of part or all of my body for medical purposes, authorize an autopsy, and direct the disposition of my remains, to the extent permitted by law;

H. To take any other action necessary to do what I authorize here, including (but not limited to) granting any waiver or release from liability required by any hospital, physician, or other health care provider; signing any documents relating to refusals of treatment or the leaving of a facility against medical advice; and pursuing any legal action in my name at the expense of my estate to force compliance with my wishes as determined by my Agent, or to seek actual or punitive damages for the failure to comply.

Section 5—My Instructions About End-of-Life Treatment

The subject of end-of-life treatment is particularly important to many people. In this paragraph, you can give general or specific instructions on the subject. The different paragraphs are options—choose only one, or write your desires or instructions in your own words (in the last option). If you are satisfied with your agent's knowledge of your values and wishes and you do not want to include instructions in the form, initial the first option and do not give instructions in the form.

Any instructions you give here will guide your agent. If you do not appoint an agent, they will guide any health care providers or surrogate decision makers who must make a decision for you if you cannot do so yourself. The instruction choices in the form describe different treatment goals you may prefer, depending on your condition.

Write the directive in your own words. If you would like to state your wishes about end-of-life treatment in your own words instead of choosing one of the options provided, you can do so in this section. Since people sometimes have different opinions on whether nutrition and hydration should be refused or stopped under certain circumstances, be sure to address this issue clearly in your directive. Nutrition and hydration means food and fluids given through a nasogastric tube or tube into your stomach, intestines, or veins, and does not include nonintrusive methods such as spoonfeeding or moistening of lips and mouth.

Some states allow the stopping of nutrition and hydration only if you expressly authorize it. If you are creating your own directive, and you do not want nutrition and hydration, state so clearly.

Health Care Advance Directive
Part II
Instructions About Health Care

5. MY INSTRUCTIONS ABOUT END-OF-LIFE TREATMENT

(Initial only ONE of the following statements)

_____ NO SPECIFIC INSTRUCTIONS. My agent knows my values and wishes, so I do not wish to include any specific instructions here.

DIRECTIVE TO WITHHOLD OR WITHDRAW TREATMENT. Although I greatly value life, I also believe that at some point, life has such diminished value that medical treatment should be stopped, and I should be allowed to die. Therefore, I do not want to receive treatment, including nutrition and hydration, when the treatment will not give me a meaningful quality of life. I do not want my life prolonged . . .

_____ . . . if the treatment will leave me in a condition of permanent unconsciousness, such as with an irreversible coma or a persistent vegetative state.

_____ . . . if the treatment will leave me with no more than some consciousness and in an irreversible condition of complete, or nearly complete, loss of ability to think or communicate with others.

_____ . . . if the treatment will leave me with no more than some ability to think or communicate with others, and the likely risks and burdens of treatment outweigh the expected benefits. Risks, burdens, and benefits include consideration of length of life, quality of life, financial costs, and my personal dignity and privacy.

_____ DIRECTIVE TO RECEIVE TREATMENT. I want my life to be prolonged as long as possible, no matter what my quality of life.

_____ DIRECTIVE ABOUT END-OF-LIFE TREATMENT IN MY OWN WORDS:

_____

_____

_____

_____

_____

Section 6—*Any Other Health Care Instructions or Limitations or Modifications of My Agent's Powers*

In this section, you can provide instructions about other health care issues that are not end-of-life treatment or nutrition and hydration. For example, you might want to include your wishes about issues like nonemergency surgery, elective medical treatments, or admission to a nursing home. Again, be careful in these instructions not to place limitations on your agent that you do not intend. For example, while you may not want to be admitted to a nursing home, placing such a restriction may make things impossible for your agent if other options are not available.

You also may limit your agent's powers in any way you wish. For example, you can instruct your agent to refuse any specific types of treatment that are against your religious beliefs or unacceptable to you for any other reasons. These might include blood transfusions, electroconvulsive therapy, sterilization, abortion, amputation, psychosurgery, or admission to a mental institution, etc. Some states limit your agent's authority to consent to or refuse some of these procedures, regardless of your health care advance directive.

Be very careful about stating limitations, because the specific circumstances surrounding future health care decisions are impossible to predict. If you do not want any limitations, simply write in "No limitations."

Section 7—Protection of Third Parties Who Rely on My Agent

In most states, health care providers cannot be forced to follow the directions of your agent if they object. However, most states also require providers to help transfer you to another provider who is willing to honor your instructions. To encourage compliance with the health care advance directive, this paragraph states that providers who rely in good faith on the agent's statements and decisions will not be held civilly liable for their actions.

Section 8—Donation of Organs at Death

In this section you can state your intention to donate bodily organs and tissues at death. If you do not wish to be an organ donor, initial the first option. The second option is a donation of any or all organs or parts. The third option allows you to donate only those organs or tissues you specify. Consider mentioning the heart, liver, lungs, kidneys, pancreas, intestine, corneas, bone, skin, heart valves, tendons, ligaments, and saphenous vein in the leg. Finally, you may limit the use of your organs by crossing out any of the four purposes listed that you do not want (transplant, therapy, research, or education). If you do not cross out any of these options, your organs may be used for any of these purposes.

---

6. ANY OTHER HEALTH CARE INSTRUCTIONS OR LIMITATIONS OR MODIFICATIONS OF MY AGENT'S POWERS

_____

_____

_____

_____

_____

7. PROTECTION OF THIRD PARTIES WHO RELY ON MY AGENT

No person who relies in good faith upon any representations by my Agent or Alternate Agent(s) shall be liable to me, my estate, my heirs or assigns, for recognizing the Agent's authority.

Upon my death (Initial one):

_____ I do not wish to donate any organs or tissue, OR
_____ I give any needed organs, tissues, or parts, OR
_____ I give only the following organs, tissues, or parts
(please specify):

_____

_____

My gift (if any) is for the following purposes (Cross out any of the following you do not want):

—Transplant
—Research
—Therapy
—Education

_____

_____

Section 9—Nomination of Guardian

Appointing a health care agent helps to avoid a court-appointed guardian for health care decision making. However, if a court becomes involved for any reason, this paragraph expressly names your agent to serve as guardian. A court does not have to follow your nomination, but normally it honors your wishes unless there is good reason to override your choice.

Section 10—Administrative Provisions

These items address miscellaneous matters that could affect the implementation of your health care advance directive.

Signing the Document

Required state procedures for signing this kind of document vary. Some require only a signature, while others have very detailed witnessing requirements. Some states simply require notarization.

The procedure in this book is likely to be far more complex than your state law requires because it combines the formal requirements from virtually every state. Follow it if you do not know your state's requirements and you want to meet the signature requirements of virtually every state.

First, sign and date the document in the presence of two witnesses—*not* your agents—and a notary.

---

9. NOMINATION OF GUARDIAN

If a guardian of my person should for any reason need to be appointed, I nominate my Agent (or his or her alternate then authorized to act), named above.

10. ADMINISTRATIVE PROVISIONS

(All apply)

—I revoke any prior health care advance directive.
—This health care advance directive is intended to be valid in any jurisdiction in which it is presented.
—A copy of this advance directive is intended to have the same effect as the original.

SIGNING THE DOCUMENT

BY SIGNING HERE I INDICATE THAT I UNDERSTAND THE CONTENTS OF THIS DOCUMENT AND THE EFFECT OF THIS GRANT OF POWERS TO MY AGENT.

I sign my name to this Health Care Advance Directive on this

_____ day of _____, _____.

My signature _____

My name _____

My current home address _____

_____

Choosing Your Witnesses

Your witnesses should know your identity personally and be able to declare that you appear to be of sound mind and under no duress or undue influence.

In order to meet the different witnessing requirements of most states, do not have the following people witness your signature:

- anyone you have chosen to make health care decisions on your behalf (agent or alternate agents)
- your treating physician, health care provider, health facility operator, or an employee of any of these
- insurers or employees of your life/health insurance provider
- anyone financially responsible for your health care costs
- anyone related to you by blood, marriage, or adoption
- anyone entitled to any part of your estate under an existing will or by operation of law, or anyone who will benefit financially from your death (your creditors should not serve as witnesses)

If you are in a nursing home or other institution, a few states have additional witnessing requirements. This form does not include witnessing language for this situation. Contact a patient advocate or an ombudsman to find out about the state's requirements in these cases.

Second, have your signature notarized. Some states permit notarization as an alternative to witnessing. Doing both witnessing and notarization is more than most states require, but doing both will meet the execution requirements of most states. This form includes a typical notary statement, but it is wise to check state law in case it requires a special form of notary acknowledgment.

WITNESS STATEMENT

I declare that the person who signed or acknowledged this document is personally known to me, that he/she signed or acknowledged this health care advance directive in my presence, and that he/she appears to be of sound mind and under no duress, fraud, or undue influence.

I am not:

—the person appointed as agent by this document,
—the principal's health care provider,
—an employee of the principal's health care provider,
—financially responsible for the principal's health care,
—related to the principal by blood, marriage, or adoption, and,
—to the best of my knowledge, a creditor of the principal or entitled to any part of his/her estate under a will now existing or by operation of law.

Witness # 1:
Signature _____ Date _____

Print Name _____

Telephone _____

Residence Address _____

Witness #2:

Signature _____ Date _____

Print Name _____

Telephone _____

Residence Address _____

NOTARIZATION

STATE OF _____

COUNTY OF _____

_____ day of _____, _____.

The said _____, known to me (or satisfactorily proven) to be the person named in the foregoing instrument, personally appeared before me, a Notary Public, within and for the State and County aforesaid, and acknowledged that he or she freely and voluntarily executed the same for the purposes stated therein.

My Commission Expires: _____

NOTARY PUBLIC

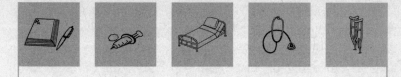

PART TWO

The Top Ten Risks: How to Understand and Avoid Them

Because most hospitals are organized along the same lines, the same kinds of problems tend to crop up over and over again in just about every hospital. And a relative handful of risks account for most of the serious injuries.

These risks are well known to researchers and health experts. Over the years, hospitals have spent billions of dollars on programs to reduce or eliminate them, with mixed results.

No matter how many checks and balances are devised to prevent these errors, hospital staffs still run up against the same fundamental problems: too much work and not enough time. False assumptions. Long hours. Tedious, repetitive work that can cause attention to wander. New people constantly coming into the workforce who don't yet have the knowledge and judgment to make the right decisions. And above all, little margin for error. Nurses, for example, perform hundreds of different tasks in a shift. Even if they do their job with 99 percent accuracy, you could still expect each one to make several errors a day. Most will be harmless, but not all.

By focusing on just these top risks, you can significantly improve your odds. In this section, we take a closer look at each of them and offer practical ways you can protect yourself.

9
Medication Errors

Everyone works hard to avoid medication errors, yet they remain the most common cause of serious injuries in the hospital.

Most medication errors are a result of lack of attention, not lack of knowledge. Chances are, the physician, pharmacist, and nurses are familiar with drugs you're taking (and they'll probably be extra careful if they're giving you anything new or unfamiliar). The problem is that they can become *too* familiar—falling into a set routine and not paying enough attention to what's going on.

It's sort of like what happens if you drive to work the same way every day. The route becomes so familiar that you stop noticing it. And if something changes—say, a new stop sign goes up—it's easy to drive by without noticing.

Dispensing medications is a tedious job. There are lots of medications, many similar in appearance and name.

Different dosages. Patients come and go, so there's not much time to learn what they're taking or why. To make matters worse, doctors need to change patients' medications all the time.

In this environment, nobody's in a better position to keep you safe than you (and your advocate). You're the last stop on the line. No drug should go into your body until you're satisfied that it's the right one.

Before You Go

If you have time, take these steps before you go to the hospital.

Make a List of All Your Medications

List everything you're taking, including:

- All *prescription* medications, including name (brand name and generic, if available—see the pharmacy label), the prescribed dosage (for example, two 50-mg tablets four times a day), and what you've *actually* been taking. Don't forget birth control pills, which become less effective when combined with some medications, and which can interfere with some treatments.
- All *nonprescription* medications, including drugs such as aspirin, ibuprofen, Tylenol, and so on. Include the name and dosage.
- All dietary supplements, vitamins, and so on.

- All herbal or natural remedies. They may interfere with drugs you'll be receiving in the hospital, or could mask or mimic symptoms.
- All alternative medicines you are taking, such as homeopathic preparations.

Also mention all allergies, especially drug allergies such as to penicillin or aspirin, and any side effects or unusual reactions you've experienced when taking medications, now or in the past.

If you don't have time to assemble this information, just put all your pill bottles in a bag and bring them with you to the hospital.

It's important to be as complete as you can (if you forget, tell the nurse or doctor about it as soon as you remember). The hospital staff doesn't know what you're taking unless you tell them. Don't assume your doctor has provided this information. Everyone needs to know what you've been taking and what might be in your system already.

Be Complete and Honest

There's something about medication regimens that can make otherwise competent adults act like guilty six-year-olds who just broke Mommy's favorite vase. If you haven't been following your medication schedule properly, don't try to cover it up. If you've been skipping doses for any reason, or if you sometimes double up on a prescription, tell your caregivers when they ask about your medications. Don't worry or be embarrassed: Nobody's going to call the prescription police. But the doctors and nurses need to know. Otherwise they may assume a certain medication isn't working as it should and needlessly take you off of it or change the dosage.

The same goes for everything else you put into your body. Many people who take homeopathic or herbal remedies don't tell their doctors, because they're afraid the doctor will get mad at them. It's true that many doctors take a dim view of such remedies, but it's your body and you can do whatever you want with it. However, if you hide the fact that you're taking other remedies, you could be putting your health at risk.

If you smoke, drink alcohol, use drugs like marijuana or cocaine, or take prescription drugs that weren't prescribed to you, let your doctor know. (The doctor is required by law to keep such information confidential.)

Be honest about your diet, too. If you're supposed to be on a low-sodium diet, but you're sneaking hot dogs and fries, come clean with your doctor. Otherwise, the doctor may think your drugs aren't working and switch them.

We're certainly not advocating that you indulge in unhealthy vices (especially against your doctor's orders), but when you're going into the hospital, the important thing is for doctors and nurses to know what's been going on in your body.

It's amazing how many people can't bring themselves to admit that they're smoking, or cheating on their diet, or doing other things they think the doctor won't approve of. Often, it seems, they're really having trouble admitting it to *themselves*. People don't like to think less of themselves, and they often go to great lengths to rationalize their behavior: "I cheated only a couple of times" (well, really a couple of times a week) or "I used to smoke marijuana, but I've pretty much quit" (except for nights and weekends).

Here's a tip that may help you come clean: *We*—your doctors, nurses, and other caregivers—*don't care if you've been bad.* We're not your mother, or your parole officer, or your priest. We're not going to call the police, or your employer, or your spouse. It's not our job to pass judgment. It's our job to help you get well. But to do that, we need accurate and complete information.

Not every piece of information is relevant, of course. If you're going in for knee surgery, for example, it may not matter much whether your cholesterol is under control. But let your caregivers sort that out—simply provide complete answers to the questions they ask.

In the Hospital

When you're admitted, a nurse will ask about the medications you're taking. If you have the list, give it to him or her. If you don't have the list or the medications, provide as much information as you can. Later, you can have someone at home or your doctor's office check your medications and you can update the list.

Don't Take Pills from Home

When you're in the hospital, don't take pills you bring from home. The hospital will give you all the medications you should be taking—including, in most cases, the same drugs you've been getting—but they'll be dispensed from the hospital pharmacy. If you also took your pills from home, you'd be getting *twice* the dosage you should.

Just to be sure, ask your nurse if your current medications are being continued, whether there have been dose changes, and what is being added to your current medication regimen. If your medication regimen is changed, ask why and what will take the place of the medications you've been getting.

Know What You're Taking and Why

When you see your doctor, tell him or her you want to know the names of each medication you're getting and why you're taking it. If the medications or dosages are different from those you take at home, ask why the change was made.

Make sure that the nurses know and understand the drug regimen that the doctor has prescribed, and that their understanding matches your understanding. For example, fluids should be given before certain chemotherapy drugs to help protect your kidneys from damage from the drugs. If the doctor explained that you'll be getting fluids but a nurse tells you they're not necessary, don't let him or her administer the chemotherapy drug. Nurses may not understand the significance of what the doctor has ordered, so it's important that you understand exactly what the doctor wants and why.

Of course, it's not easy to challenge your nurse if you think he or she's doing something wrong. But it's worth the effort, because the stakes are high. In Chapter 3, we discussed some strategies on how to get the nurses to be your allies instead of adversaries. You can stand your ground without being confrontational.

For example, here's how you might handle the preceding situation:

NURSE: Okay, Mr. Herbert, we're going to be giving you some IV medications.

PATIENT: Is that my chemotherapy?

NURSE: Yes, it is.

PATIENT: May I ask you a question?

NURSE: Of course.

PATIENT: The doctor told me that I should be getting lots of IV fluids with this drug to protect my kidneys.

NURSE: He never said it to me. That's not how we do it here.

PATIENT: Well, maybe you can help me understand. These drugs can be hard on the kidneys, can't they?

NURSE: Yes, they can.

PATIENT: I'd rather be safe than sorry. You can understand my concern, can't you?

NURSE: Yes, but there's nothing about in on the chart. (Taking the patient's arm) I'm sure it's fine.

PATIENT (gently pulling arm away): Maybe. But could you check with the doctor first?

NURSE: It's after office hours.

PATIENT: But it's important that I start the treatment right away, right? So is there a way to get in touch with him?

NURSE: Well, he may not call back right away. But if

you're willing to wait until he calls . . .

PATIENT: I would feel a lot better about it. Thanks.

Check Your Records

Ask the nurse to show you the medication orders on the chart so you can check them for accuracy. It's easy to make mistakes—many medications have similar names, or dosages may be entered incorrectly. Any mistakes can cause a chain reaction of medication errors during your entire stay.

First, be sure orders are legible. Have the nurse point out where the doctor's orders for medications are included. If you can't read the doctor's handwriting, can you be sure the nurse and pharmacy can read it correctly? One of the most common causes of medication errors is illegible handwriting on the prescription. Pay special attention to the dosage. The most common type of medication error is administering the incorrect dosage.

Drugs may be listed by their generic names, not their trade names. If you're not sure, ask whether they're the same. (For example, the blood thinner warfarin is often referred to by its trade name, Coumadin.)

Each medication order should include:

- The name of the medication.
- The dosage, usually in milligrams (mg)—10 mg, 50 mg.
- The route of administration. For example, p.o. stands for *"per os,"* Latin for "by mouth." IM stands for "intramuscular"—injected into the muscle. IV means "intravenous"—

introduced by a needle into your veins. Usually, it is assumed that the drugs are taken by mouth unless noted otherwise.

- The frequency of the dose.

ABBREVIATIONS USED ON CHARTS AND PRESCRIPTIONS

Most abbreviations are based on Latin, a throwback to the days when it was the common language of medicine.

ac = *ante cibum;* before meals

b.i.d. = *bis in die;* two times a day

c̄ = *cum;* with

caps. = capsule

gtt. = *guttae;* drop

h = *hora;* hour

h.s. = *hora somni;* bedtime

IM = intramuscular; injected into the muscle

IV = intravenous; introduced through a needle into a vein

NPO = *nulla per os;* nothing by mouth

o.d. = *oculus dexter;* right eye

o.s. = *oculus sinister;* left eye

o.u. = *oculus uterque;* each eye

p.c. = *post cibum;* after meals

p.o. = *per os;* by mouth

prn = *pro re nata;* as needed

q. = *quaque;* every

q.d. = *quaque die;* every day

q.h. = *quaque hora;* every hour

q.i.d. = *quater in die;* four times a day

q2h = every two hours

t.i.d. = *ter in die;* three times a day

R = rectal

sl or SL = sublingual; given under the tongue—for example, a dissolving lozenge

sq = subcutaneous; injected just under the skin

T = topical; applied to the skin—for example, an ointment

Ask About Drug Interactions

If you're receiving more than one drug at a time (as most hospitalized patients do), ask the nurse whether the pharmacy has checked for drug interactions—that is, whether the drugs will combine in harmful ways. Some drugs block the effects of others, some make other drugs more potent. Some drugs should never be taken together, as they can combine in potentially deadly ways. Most pharmacies have a computer program that automatically flags dangerous combinations.

Be sure they recheck for interactions if any medications are added during your stay.

To make sure, you can check on drug interactions yourself. Have a friend check them out with your local pharmacist for any potential contraindications. Or consult a drug guide such as *The Pill Book.* Or ask the nurses; they usually have professional guides listing drug interactions. You or your advocate can call the hospital pharmacist also; that's a great resource. Simply call the hospital switchboard and ask for the hospital pharmacy department. When you get the pharmacy, explain who you are and what you'd like to know.

If your medications change, be sure *everybody* knows. If you have several doctors, make sure they know what the other doctors are prescribing. For example, if one doctor changes your medications, make sure to tell all other doctors and your nurse. Don't assume they checked the chart.

When It's Time for Your Medications

The most critical time for preventing medication errors is when the nurse shows up to give them to you. Here are some steps to keep you safe.

Make Your Own Checklist

Hospitals use checklists all the time to prevent errors. You can too.

You don't need to be an expert on every drug you're getting. The main thing is to be sure you're getting the right medications, in the right amounts, at the right time.

You or your advocate can bring a pen and notebook, and keep it by your hospital bed. Ask your nurse for a list of your medications and when you should be taking them.

Write down each medication in your notebook, one per page. Write the name at the top, then the dosage and frequency of administration, what the medication is for, and what you may expect to feel when you take it. When your nurse brings the medications the first time, ask him or her to show you which are which and make a note of what they look like in your notebook—for example, "small white pill, triangle shaped."

Keep your notebook handy. Whenever you're due for your medications, use it to make sure you're getting the right drug at the right time. Under each medication, write down the time and dosage.

Watch for Unexpected Changes in Routines

An unexpected change is a warning sign of trouble. If something happens that differs from what you expect, *ask why*. For example, if you've been getting a pill once a day and the nurse brings you a second dose, ask if the dosage was changed and why.

If They Do Make a Mistake

If you know or suspect that you received a wrong medicine, tell someone as soon as possible. Make sure the error is noted in your chart and ask your doctor about it when you see him or her. Be alert for side effects.

When You're Ready to Leave

When you're ready to leave the hospital, ask the nurse to go over each medication you'll be taking at home, including the name of the drug, what it's for, the dosage, and any precautions or side effects to watch out for. You should receive written instructions as well. Update your medication list from home if there are any changes.

Riskiest Types of Errors

Many medication errors are fairly harmless—for example, if you miss a dose or get an extra dose of a drug that's being discontinued.

Put most of your attention on the types of errors that can cause the most harm. Here are the big ones.

Wrong Medication

Most hospitals use something called the "unit-dose" system for administering medications. The pharmacy figures out what you should be taking and when, and sends up a tray to the nursing station with everybody's medication sorted into individual little cups or containers. It's a proven way to cut down on medication errors, because the doses are prepared by a pharmacist away from the hustle and bustle of the hospital floor. And it works great— as long as the right cup gets to the right patient. But if you've recently been moved to a new room or bed, if you're sharing a room, or if there's someone else in the hospital with a similar name, you may get someone else's medication. And, of course, that also means you didn't get yours.

The first line of defense: *Make sure that the person giving you the medication knows your name.* It's not enough that the nurses talk to you about your grandkids and come in and out of your room every ten minutes. They could do all that and still think you're Mrs. Miller down the hall. When they're coming around with the medication chart, make sure they check your ID bracelet against the medication sheet before giving any medications. This is the best way to be sure the right medication is getting to the right patient. The nurse should take the medication sheet to the bedside with the medicine in hand, ask your name, and check your response against the name on the medication sheet.

The nurse should ask if you have any allergies—*every* time you receive your medication. Even if the nurse has given you the medication ten times already, he or she should ask. Many patients suddenly remember they do in fact have a drug allergy. You should also have an allergy band on your arm next to your hospital ID bracelet; it should be checked with each medication administration.

If the nurse doesn't address you by name, make sure he or she checks your identification bracelet before giving you medications. That's especially important if it's not your regular nurse. If he or she doesn't check, simply say, "I just want to make sure I'm getting the right medications. I'm Betty Jones."

Even if you're getting the right medicine cup, the medicines may still be wrong. Pharmacists make mistakes too—putting Mrs. Miller's medications in your cup, for example, or misreading the medication name or dosage, or simply pulling the wrong bottle of pills off the shelf. So your second line of defense is to pull out that notebook you prepared and make sure every medication in the cup matches what you wrote down.

Too Much Medication

This is an especially big problem for drugs that have to be reconstituted—for example, a powder that has to be mixed with water to create an injectable liquid—and drugs that have to be diluted in an IV solution. If someone miscalculates the amount of fluid required or reads the instructions wrong, you could get an overdose. And not just a slight overdose—a misplaced decimal point could result in your getting ten or a hundred times the intended dose. Overdoses can also occur from double dosing, although with unit dose systems, that's less likely to occur.

Unfortunately, as a patient you're not in a good position to tell whether a drug was reconstituted properly before it's given to you. But try to listen to what your body is telling you. If you've had the drug before, pay special attention to anything that seems different or unusual. Did you feel an excessive amount of pain or burning when the drug was injected or introduced into your IV line? Does the drug make you disoriented, dizzy, or nauseous? If you feel any adverse or unusual reactions at all, *tell your nurse immediately, and say that you think it might be related to the drug you received.*

Getting Medications for Too Long

Make sure you're not getting medications after your doctor has discontinued them.

When the doctor discontinues a drug you've been getting, he or she writes the order in your chart. But sometimes the word doesn't get to the pharmacy in time. Sometimes it doesn't get there at all. Or the order may be misunderstood or overlooked. Again, use your notebook: Once the doctor or nurse tells you a drug has been discontinued, you should put a big X through it.

If the nurse brings you a drug that's been discontinued, you need to take two steps: Refuse to take it, and ask the nurse to make sure the pharmacy knows it's supposed to be discontinued. Without this second step, the drug will keep showing up, and you may not notice it next time.

IMPORTANT THINGS TO KNOW ABOUT YOUR MEDICATION

- its name
- what it looks like
- what it is used for and why you are taking it; many medicines have multiple uses
- how often it is to be given
- how it is administered—by mouth, IV, rectally, under the tongue, intramuscular injection, topically (i.e., applied to the skin)
- possible side effects
- potential interactions with other drugs, food, herbs, and vitamins, and whether they need to be given at different times to prevent interactions

10

Side Effects of Drugs

All drugs have potential side effects. But a handful are especially dangerous. Make sure you're paying extra attention to your medications if you're receiving any of the following:

- antibiotics, especially aminoglycosides
- cancer medications
- heart medications

Many of these drugs have what doctors call a "narrow therapeutic window." In plain English, that means drugs for which the *effective* dose (the dose needed to treat your illness) is close to the *toxic* dose (the dose that can cause you harm). Some drugs have a wide therapeutic window—even a significant overdose isn't likely to cause you long-term harm. Others, such as cancer drugs, have a very narrow therapeutic window, or sometimes none at all—the dose you need to treat the disease is likely to make you sick. The narrower the therapeutic window, the less margin for error and the greater the need for monitoring.

If you're taking high-risk drugs, you need to be extra vigilant to be sure that (1) you're getting the right drugs and dosage, and (2) you really need to be taking them.

Ask the doctor:

- How are these drugs being monitored for toxicity?
- What part of the body is most likely to be affected by side effects—for example, can they cause liver damage? Kidney damage? Hearing loss or visual changes? Dizziness or vertigo?
- What side effects or warning signs should I be aware of?
- How long will I have to take them?
- What special precautions should be followed—by me and by the nursing staff—to reduce the risk of ill effects?

Antibiotics

Even if you're not allergic to them, antibiotics can be dangerous. Unnecessary antibiotics can provoke secondary infections, especially in hospitals, where germs abound. Ask your doctor about any antibiotic prescription—why you're taking it, what are the potential dangers, and whether it's absolutely necessary to begin it immediately or whether you can wait.

Aminoglycosides

These drugs are a class of antibiotics with risks all

their own. They're very powerful and are often used when infections are resistant to ordinary antibiotics (because so many antibiotics are used in hospitals, they tend to become breeding grounds for drug-resistant infections).

If you're being treated for infection—especially a resistant infection—ask your doctor or nurse whether you're receiving an aminoglycoside. Streptomycin, tobramycin, and gentamicin are examples of aminoglycosides.

When these drugs are given *topically* (that is, applied to the skin as an ointment or cream), they're reasonably safe. However, ear drops can cause ear nerve damage and hearing loss. It doesn't happen often, but it does occur, especially in patients who are older or very young.

With aminoglycosides, the pharmacist is very much a part of your care. He or she may be monitoring your blood levels and ordering medication dose changes based on the blood levels. Ask if the pharmacists are involved in your medication monitoring and talk with them if you have questions. Be sure to ask who is monitoring the blood levels and prescribing the doses. Find out when blood levels will be checked. If the schedule isn't followed, stop and ask questions.

The length of time you'll need these drugs varies according to blood levels and severity of infection. When these drugs are used, the infection is usually resistant to everything else available.

When taken internally, aminoglycosides have a high risk of causing nerve damage. The result can be deafness or blindness. They need to be monitored to be sure they don't build up to toxic levels, and they need to be used for only short periods of time.

The exact length of therapy depends on the infection, but therapy that lasts more than ten days has a higher risk of nerve damage.

If your doctor orders an aminoglycoside, be sure that he or she is checking your blood levels at least every twenty-four to seventy-two hours to be sure the drugs aren't building up to toxic levels in your bloodstream.

Find out how long the treatment should last, and make yourself a big reminder in your notebook of what the last day should be. If the nurse brings you the drug after that day, refuse to take it and demand that the doctor and pharmacy be notified immediately. *Even a single extra day can result in severe and permanent damage.*

Cancer Medicines

Most cancer medicines are extremely toxic. Not only can they make you sick when you take them, but they also can cause lasting damage and increase your risk of cancer later on. Even a mild overdose can be dangerous. *Be sure that the people who administer these drugs know what they're doing and take time to do it right.* If you have any doubts on either count, you may want to refuse the drugs until you talk to your doctor.

Be alert for signs of toxicity or side effects with these drugs, such as pain or burning sensations, rashes or soreness. For example, if you're receiving the drug cisplatin, loss of taste or a tingling sensation in the fingers, toes, or face are signs of toxicity. Have the nurse inform the doctor immediately; he or she may discontinue the drug to avoid permanent damage.

Also be watchful for signs of infection. Many of these drugs can hurt your immune system temporarily, leaving you more open to infection.

Heart Medications

Heparin, warfarin (Coumadin), digoxin, and many other blood pressure and heart anti-arrhythmic drugs can build up in your system. If you feel weak or dizzy, let your nurse know immediately. Blood thinners such as warfarin and heparin make you more prone to bruising and bleeding. Be sure your levels are being monitored closely to avoid toxicity.

Allergies

If you know you're allergic to certain kinds of drugs, tell your doctor and nurse. Any allergies should be noted on your chart (and often are prominently noted with a colorful sticker as well), yet many errors continue to occur because someone—the nurse, pharmacist, or physician—didn't realize the patient had an allergy or didn't realize that a drug contained an allergic ingredient. Be sure that anything else you are allergic to is added to your allergy band—i.e. bee stings, strawberries, eggs, peanuts, etc.

A rash is considered an adverse reaction, not a true allergy. It may be uncomfortable but is seldom dangerous. In many cases an antihistamine may be given to treat the rash—especially if the drug is needed for treatment and no good alternatives exist. Rashes are sometimes caused by the illness, not the drug.

True allergic reactions involve swelling, difficulty breathing, blood pressure changes, heart irregularities, and/or welts and hives. They can be life threatening if the swelling closes up your breathing passages. Fortunately, their effects can be reversed if they're caught in time.

The most common drug allergies involve antibiotics and aspirin-related drugs, including antiarthritis drugs such as Motrin and Vioxx. Tylenol (acetaminophen) is safe to give to someone with aspirin allergies.

The best defense: If you know you have allergies, remind the nurse whenever you're given a new or unfamiliar medication. Tell him or her, "I have allergies; will that be a problem with this medicine?"

Also be on guard yourself for any potentially allergic drugs.

- If you're allergic to penicillin, also watch for any drugs in the penicillin class (such as V-Cillin, amoxicillin, etc.). Also beware of *cephalosporin* antibiotics (such as Keflex, Ceftin, Cefzil, and Omnicef). These drugs are chemical cousins to the penicillins and sometimes cause the same kind of reactions in people who are allergic to penicillin.
- If you're allergic to aspirin, you need to avoid most other types of nonsteroidal anti-inflammatory drugs (NSAIDs), such as ibuprofen (Motrin or Advil) and Celebrex. Aceta-

minophen (Tylenol) should be safe. Other drugs may have aspirin or aspirin-related drugs as an ingredient. Darvocet of any form has aspirin properties. This is a frequently used pain medication.

MEDICATIONS TO WATCH IF YOU HAVE DRUG ALLERGIES

If you're allergic to penicillin, watch out for:

PENICILLINS

Common drug names include amoxicillin, ampicillin, Augmentin, bicillin, Pen-Vee-K, piperacillin, Principen, procaine penicillin, Trimox.

CEPHALOSPORINS

These are chemical cousins to the penicillins and work in a similar fashion. People who are allergic to penicillin are more likely to be allergic to cephalosporins, and vice versa. Common cephalosporins include Ceclor, Cedax, Cefobid, Ceftin, Cefzil, Claforan, Duricef, Fortaz, Keflex, Kefzol, Maxipime, Mefoxin, Omnicef, Rocephin, Suprax, Tazidime, Vantin, Velosef, Zinacef.

SAFE ALTERNATIVES

Erythromycin, clarithromycin (Biaxin), azithromycin (Zithromax), Dynabac, E.E.S., ERYC, EryPed, Ery-Tab, PCE, Pediazole

Sulfa, Bactrim, Septra

Tetracyclines: doxycycline, Minocin, Sumycin, Vibramycin, Vibra-Tabs

Quinolones: Avelox, Cipro, Floxin, levoquin, mazaquin, Tequin

If you're allergic to aspirin, watch out for:

aspirin
Darvocet
Motrin, Advil (ibuprofen)
Celebrex

SAFE ALTERNATIVES:
bextra, Tylenol, Ultram

Other allergy-prone drugs

Iodine, found in dyes used for X-ray studies of the bowel, digestive system, and the arteries. Depending on the type of reaction you have and the tests you need, you may be given *antihistamines* before the test is performed to avoid an allergic reaction to the iodine. If so, be sure that everyone around you knows this is occurring, and an anaphylactic kit and emergency kit are at your bedside with qualified nursing personnel to administer the medications. Remember this: Seafood such as shrimp and lobster contain iodine.

11

Infection

Hospitals are home to the toughest germs, because hospitals handle the sickest of the sick. Over the years, as germs have been exposed to the drugs used in hospitals, many have evolved into *drug-resistant* varieties that are immune to ordinary antibiotics.

Some 5 to 10 percent of hospitalized patients develop infections. Teaching hospitals, which tend to treat the sickest patients of all, usually have the highest rates of infection. Many of these infections are resistant even to the most powerful medications. That's why it's important to avoid infection if you can.

All hospitals have infection control departments, which are responsible for preventing hospital infections and controlling outbreaks if they do occur. Yet the most effective infection control procedures are pretty simple. The hard part is getting people to follow them consistently. That's where you can really help yourself.

Types of Infections

There are three types of infections: bacterial, fungal, and viral.

Bacterial

Most hospital infections are bacterial and are treated with antibiotics. However, the infections found in hospitals are often resistant to ordinary antibiotics and require stronger drugs.

The key to good treatment is a good diagnosis. If the bacteria aren't properly identified, you probably won't get the right drugs. Delays in proper treatment can be life threatening.

An increasingly common hospital infection is methicillin-resistant *Staphylococcus aureus* (MRSA). It's a very nasty infection and hard to get rid of, and it's common in hospitals and nursing homes. As the name implies, it's resistant to the antibiotics used to treat other staph infections; it requires more powerful (and dangerous) drugs such as vancomycin. Recently, strains of MRSA have emerged that are resistant even to this drug.

MRSA is difficult to eliminate from the hospital environment. It's spread primarily on the hands of hospital personnel—one more reason to insist that the people who care for you wash their hands.

Before you go into the hospital, you can call its infection control department and ask about MRSA. Though it's a problem in most hospitals, it's epidemic in some.

Nontuberculous mycobacteria (NTM) are also common in hospitals. Evidence suggests that NTM outbreaks may be on the rise. One theory is that reduced hot-water temperatures may be partly to blame. NTMs are often mistaken for other kinds of infections, but they require different treatments. So if you do get infected and treatment doesn't seem to be helping, ask whether you've been screened for NTMs.

Fungal

Invasive aspergillosis (IA) is a fungal infection. The spores that cause it are common in hospitals, but usually they don't cause widespread outbreaks. You're at increased risk of IA if your immune system is impaired by disease or by treatment (for example, many cancer medications). Another fungal infection, candidiasis (so-called yeast infection), can infect you if your immune system is compromised. These skin infections can grow when your skin is moist from sweat and folded over on itself.

Fungal infections can be carried on the air, and an effective way to prevent them is by maintaining good air quality in the hospital. The Centers for Disease Control has published guidelines that all hospitals should follow.

Viral

Viruses account for about 5 percent of hospital infections. Depending on the type of virus, the doctor may prescribe antiviral drugs. Antibiotics are ineffective for viral infection; in fact, they can actually leave you more susceptible to other infections. A secondary bacterial infection can easily occur as a complication of a viral infection. In such cases, of course, antibiotics are used to treat the secondary infection.

Strategies Before You Go In

There are some steps you can take before you go to the hospital that can help avoid, or at least combat, these infections.

Eat and drink. You're at greater risk for infection if you're malnourished or dehydrated. Even if you're not feeling well before you're admitted, try to get lots of protein and vitamins in your diet, and drink as much as you can, to keep your immune system strong. If necessary, ask your doctor about nutritional supplements such as Ensure.

Avoid depression and anxiety, or get it treated. Depression and anxiety often accompany illness, especially chronic illness. Depression, especially, is often overlooked.

Both depression and anxiety can weaken the immune system, increasing your risk of infection and complications. If you think you might be depressed, talk to your doctor and get treated for it.

Strategies in the Hospital

Most infections spread from one patient to another on the hands of health care workers. Some spread in other ways—for example, Legionnaires' disease and certain fungal infections tend to spread by way of the heating and air-conditioning systems—but they're relatively rare. Doctors and nurses are the most common source of infection, simply because they have the most hands-on contact with the most patients.

Your skin is a very effective barrier against most infections—if it's not damaged or broken. Unfortunately, skin is often broken in the hospital—by intravenous lines, surgical wounds, bedsores, or urinary catheters. And, of course, these are exactly the things that nurses are most likely to touch with their hands.

Breaking the Chain

Plain soap and water are extremely effective in stopping the spread of infection. Beginning more than a hundred years ago, hand washing was one of the first measures that hospitals took to reduce infections. It remains the most effective way to avoid infection. It's simple, natural, and free from side effects.

The challenge is to be sure that health workers wash their hands before touching your body. It's easy for people to cut corners when they're in a hurry. Some nurses may think that they don't need to wash their hands if they're only taking a quick look at your IV site. The fact is, any contact can transmit germs to you.

Overall, health care workers in hospitals wash their hands only about half as often as they should. And when they do, they often don't wash them long enough to do a good job of removing germs. Though hospitals mount aggressive campaigns to improve hand washing—distributing literature, conducting classes, and giving feedback on hand-washing techniques—these efforts usually have little lasting effect.

CDC GUIDELINES FOR HAND WASHING

The Centers for Disease Control says that except in emergencies, hospital personnel should always wash their hands:

- before performing invasive procedures
- before taking care of patients whose immune systems are not working properly
- before taking care of newborns (whose immune systems are not yet fully developed)
- before and after touching wounds, whether surgical, traumatic, or associated with a device such as a catheter or intravenous line
- after situations during which microbial contamination of hands is likely to occur, especially those involving contact with mucous membranes (mouth, nose, rectum, or vagina), blood or body fluids such as mucus, phlegm, urine, stool, or drainage from a wound
- after touching supplies or devices used in collecting urine specimens or other body fluids
- after taking care of an infected patient
- between contacts with different patients in high-risk units

Most routine, brief patient-care activities, such as taking blood pressure, do not require hand washing, says the CDC, nor do most routine hospital activities involving indirect patient contact, such as handling patient medications, food, or other objects.

For routine hand washing, the CDC recommends "a vigorous rubbing together of all surfaces of lathered hands for at least 10 seconds, followed by thorough rinsing under a stream of water." Generally, plain soap should be used for hand washing unless otherwise indicated. Antimicrobial soaps should be used before caring for newborns, between patients in high-risk units, and before taking care of a patient whose immune system is failing.

To reduce your risk of getting an infection in the hospital, be sure that *everyone washes his or her hands before touching you*—especially if the person will be handling an IV line, catheter, or wound. Every time. Ideally, doctors and nurses should wash their hands in your room, immediately before they touch you, to reduce the risk of their hands getting recontaminated.

If you don't see them do it, ask them to do so—whether it's your doctor, nurse, a lab or X-ray technician. Don't be shy no matter how rushed the person seems or how minor the task seems to be. The stakes are that high.

If you notice an ongoing problem with people not washing their hands, bring up your concerns with your primary nurse or the nursing supervisor on your floor.

Keep an eye on the doctor, too. Studies suggest that doctors are even less diligent about washing their hands than nurses.

Here's an example of how you can stand your ground without alienating your nurse or doctor:

DOCTOR: (entering the room): Okay, let's take a look at that incision . . .

PATIENT: Doctor, I wonder if you could do something for me. Would you mind washing your hands first?

DOCTOR: Oh, don't worry. My hands are clean. I just need a quick peek . . .

PATIENT: It's just that I've been reading about how common hospital infections are. And from what I read, I understand that the CDC says everyone should wash their hands before they touch a wound . . .

DOCTOR: So when did you get a medical degree?

PATIENT: It's just what I read. It said hand washing is the single most important way to stop the spread of hospital infections. Did I understand it right?

DOCTOR: Well, that's the CDC's opinion. I wash my hands all the time. And none of my patients has ever had a problem.

PATIENT: I understand. Still, I'd be more comfortable if you washed your hands first. Is there any reason not to?

DOCTOR: I suppose not.

PATIENT: Thanks. It'll put my mind at ease.

Not all people who come into your room need to wash their hands—only when they are providing hands-on care. The dietary and housekeeping staff, for example, won't be washing their hands when they enter your room, because they are unlikely to be touching you.

Visitors with colds should wash their hands when they enter your room, or should avoid touching you or visiting you altogether. The common cold is much more likely to be transmitted by way of the hands than by the air.

RISK ALERT: CANCER THERAPY

Chemotherapy and radiation treatments for cancer tend to put your immune system on the fritz for a while, leaving you susceptible to infection. In addition, the disease itself may harm your immune system or create opportunities for infection to set in. In fact, infection—not cancer—is the leading cause of death among hospitalized cancer patients.

If you can, avoid being in the hospital when you're receiving or recovering from cancer treatments. If you must be in the hospital, the staff should be taking extra precautions to avoid exposing you to germs. Signs should be posted on your door requiring everyone who enters your room to wash his or her hands. To reduce the risk of infection, the nurses or doctor may insist that visitors not enter your room at all, or to wear masks. Anyone who's even slightly ill, or who has small children, shouldn't visit you. The door to your room should be kept shut to reduce the risk of germs entering.

Avoiding Equipment-Related Infections

The CDC guidelines also address infection control policies for hospital equipment. It's not possible to sterilize everything that comes into contact with a patient. The CDC says that any item that comes in contact with normally sterile tissue (such as a wound or IV site) should be sterilized.

Mucous membranes (such as the inside of the mouth and nasal passages) are generally resistant to common bacterial infections, but they may not be resistant to many other microorganisms such as viruses and tubercle bacilli (bacteria that cause tuberculosis). The CDC recommends that equipment touching mucous membranes be disinfected.

In general, intact skin acts as an effective barrier to most germs. The CDC therefore advises that items that touch only intact skin need only be clean, not sterile or disinfected.

High-Risk Categories

Urinary Tract Infections

Urinary tract infections (often referred to as UTIs in the hospital) are the most common type of hospital-acquired infection, accounting for about 40 percent of all cases. Nearly all of them are linked to the use of urinary catheters.

The risk of infection is directly related to how long the catheter is left in. The longer it's in, the greater the risk, especially after three to five days.

To prevent UTIs, avoid getting a urinary catheter if you can. Considering their role in infection, these catheters are probably overused in hospitals. Many times, catheters are inserted routinely in the emergency room and simply left in place if you're then admitted to the hospital.

Urinary catheters are often used for patients who have trouble holding their urine. For patients who are incontinent, confined to bed, or can't get to the bathroom without assistance, a urinary catheter does make nursing duties easier. In addition, there's less chance of a patient falling trying to get to the bathroom, less chance of the skin breaking down from exposure to urine, and no embarrassing "accidents" for the patient.

Ask that you not be catheterized if possible. If you can use the bathroom, a portable commode, or a bedpan, those options are preferable. (Using the commode takes less effort and is less stressful than using a bedpan, and you are better able to empty your bladder and bowels on a commode.) If you need to have your urine output monitored, it can be measured in a collection pan set inside the toilet or commode. Frequently, your urine output must be measured accurately to detect changes in kidney function. In this case, a urinary catheter is needed.

Other alternatives to a catheter:

- A condom catheter (for men). It slips over the penis rather than having a tube inserted into the bladder. This option doesn't always work very well, because the condom can easily slip off the penis, especially if the patient moves around.

- Intermittent catheterization. A sterile catheter is used only when the bladder becomes full and the patient can't urinate. This option is usually reserved for surgical patients who are trying to retrain their bladder to work (many medications given during surgery interfere with bladder function). It's also used in patients who have no nerve function in the bladder area.

If you must have a catheter, be sure your nurses handle it gently! Trauma to the urinary tract during catheter insertion, maintenance, or removal increases the risk of UTIs.

Be sure that nurses are cleaning the catheter at least every eight hours with soap and water and a warm washcloth. Mucus and germs can collect at the insertion spot and cause infection. (If you're the advocate for a patient who's disoriented, ask the nurses how often they're changing the catheter.)

Be sure that when you're sitting up in a chair or walking, the collection bag is lower than your waist level, to keep urine from backing up into the bladder and not draining freely. Be sure to keep any kinks out of the tubing as well.

If you have a urinary catheter but your bladder constantly feels full, the catheter might be kinked or clogged with mucus or blood from your bladder. Infection can result.

Your bladder can also feel full if you have bladder spasms. Spasms can be caused by the catheter irritating the urethra (the opening to the bladder), or by blood in the bladder. Tell your nurse if you're experiencing bladder spasms.

You may have a bladder infection even if you don't have symptoms. Those most susceptible are older patients, those with diabetes or nerve damage, and children. A urine test will identify infections.

Pneumonia

Pneumonia is the second most common type of infection in hospitals, and one of the most serious.

The best way to avoid pneumonia is to keep moving. That's why your nurses insist that you get up and start walking as soon as possible after your operation. Walking and activity (as well as coughing and exercises prescribed by a respiratory therapist) help the lungs clear out the phlegm where germs can hide and breed.

These measures have also been shown to help prevent pneumonia:

- Minimize the use of sedatives. These drugs make your breathing more shallow and limit your activity. That allows fluid and germs to move into your lungs. (However, you may require sedatives for other reasons; talk to your doctor.)
- Limit exposure to invasive devices, such as ventilators. The less equipment going into your throat and lungs, the less chance for contamination.
- Put the bed in a semirecumbent position—that is, with the head gently raised—instead of flat. If the head of the bed is raised, fluid is less likely to accumulate and germs from your throat are less likely to spread to your lungs.

- Avoid getting a feeding tube, if possible. And ask to have it removed as soon as possible. Feeding tubes increase the risk of pneumonia because they are invasive and often breed germs. This provides a way for them to get into your lungs and cause breathing problems. If a patient chokes on the feeding tube, the liquid is easily aspirated into the lungs, causing pneumonia to develop.

You're at increased risk for pneumonia if

- you're placed on a ventilator for more than forty-eight hours
- you're treated in the ICU
- your hospital stay is lengthy (the longer the stay, the higher the risk)

In these situations, it's especially important that you be monitored for early signs of infection and treated early and aggressively if signs of pneumonia appear.

Treatment for pneumonia depends on the organisms involved. Often it's more than one kind. Ask the doctor what types of germs are causing it and how it's being treated. Combinations of antibiotics are the treatment of choice. When a single antibiotic is used (even a so-called broad-spectrum antibiotic that works against several types of organisms), it often fails to work.

Avoiding Infections at the IV Site

An intravenous (IV) line delivers medication, fluids, and/or nutrition through a hollow needle (known as a catheter) inserted into your vein. It's connected to clear plastic tubing (the "line"). Plastic bags containing medications and fluids are connected to the tubing. Sometimes multiple bags are used, connected at various points along the tubing. The flow of medication may be controlled by a simple device attached to the line or, for greater precision, by an IV pump—a device about the size of a brick that pumps fluids through the line at a predetermined rate.

IVs are a prime source of infection among hospitalized patients, for four reasons:

- They create a break in the skin.
- The needle rests directly in the vein, creating a direct pathway for germs into the bloodstream.
- The line usually remains open for hours or days, allowing germs to multiply.
- The needle and the medication can irritate the surrounding tissue, making it less able to fight infection.

For all these reasons, pay special attention to the condition of your IV sites. Pain, irritation, redness, swelling, warmth, or tenderness to the touch may all be signs of a developing infection. Tell the nurse *immediately;* the goal is to stop the infection before it moves down into your bloodstream.

Prevention starts with proper technique when the line is first put in. Starting an IV line should be a sterile procedure. The nurse should wash his or her hands *and* wear a new pair of gloves. The site where the IV is to be inserted should be thoroughly disinfected.

After the IV is started, the site is bandaged to help

prevent infection. Most nurses use transparent dressings so that they can monitor the site for redness or swelling without removing the dressing.

Some hospitals use special IV teams to insert and monitor intravenous lines—a team of nurses who specialize in the procedure. If your hospital uses an IV team, that's a good sign that it's serious about infection control, as these teams have been shown to reduce IV-related infections and other complications.

Once the line is in, it should continue to be treated as a *sterile site*. In other words, the site itself should come into contact only with sterile surfaces. That means:

- Nurses should put on a new pair of gloves before they change the dressings or adjust the IV.
- While the dressing is off, the site must not be contaminated by coming into contact with your sheet, blanket, hospital gown, or other nonsterile surface.
- Neither you nor anyone else should touch the site while the dressing is off.
- The site should be cleansed with an antibacterial solution and a new dressing should be applied.

(Related procedures, such as drawing blood or administering shots, should also be considered sterile procedures, with the same precautions taken.)

Unfortunately, these rules are often violated in practice. For example, in my years of nursing I have witnessed nurses putting the catheter on the patient's sheet while they're prepping the site. So even though the site is sterile, the catheter that actually goes into the patient's vein has been contaminated. Similarly, I have seen nurses and others touch the spot for an IV site with their bare fingers to feel the vein after cleansing it, then insert the IV catheter without recleansing the site.

If you see your nurse engaging in such behavior, *insist that he or she immediately stop the procedure and start over with proper precautions.* If the needle has become contaminated by sitting on your bedsheet, tell the nurse to throw it away and get a new one. If the nurse dismisses your concerns, refuse to allow the procedure to go forward. If necessary, ask for a supervisor. IV-related infections can be life threatening, so the nurse's feelings have to take a backseat.

The longer you have an IV line in place, the greater the risk of infection. If the site becomes inflamed or infected, the nurse should remove the needle and notify the doctor, if necessary. If you see pus or other drainage around your IV site, it's getting infected and needs to be changed immediately. Many nurses will want to leave the IV in until the vein no longer works. That's asking for trouble. *Request that the site be changed.* Diligent nurses and IV teams are on the lookout for infection and change the IV site at the first sign of inflammation.

Blood Infections

Bloodstream infections comprise about 10 percent of all hospital-related infections.

The stakes are high for avoiding these infections. On average, they add about two weeks to the hospital stay. Even more alarming, the death rate is high—about 25 percent.

The leading cause of blood infections is IV catheters, but a blood infection is much more serious than an ordinary IV infection.

About 90 percent of all blood infections in the hospital can be traced to the use of one device: the central venous catheter (CVC). While ordinary IV lines are inserted into *peripheral* veins near the surface of the body, the central venous catheter goes directly into a *central* vein deep in the body. That means that any infection is introduced directly into the main blood supply, where it can travel quickly throughout your body.

One study found that about 5 percent of patients getting a CVC develop a potentially life-threatening blood infection. The key factor affecting the infection rate is *how long the line remains in place.* It makes no difference how often the catheter itself is replaced. Therefore, the best way to avoid this infection is to avoid having a CVC inserted at all unless and until it becomes necessary, and having it removed as soon as possible.

CVCs are inserted routinely in the critical-care unit and in the surgery department. They're used for monitoring blood pressure, heart pressures, and oxygen levels in the blood. They're also used to administer medications and blood. Be sure you understand why your catheter is needed.

The skin is the most common source of infection of CVCs. To minimize the risk of infection, CVCs should be inserted and changed under sterile conditions (see the previous section on IV lines). As with IVs, a special team helps ensure proper technique.

Once the CVC is inserted, it should be handled or

manipulated as little as possible. The insertion site must be kept meticulously clean and disinfected.

Studies suggest that where the catheter is inserted makes a difference: The subclavian site (below the collarbone) is less likely to cause infection than other sites.

CVCs are also used for total parenteral nutrition (TPN). TPN is a special type of IV solution that provides your body with all the essential nutrients and vitamins it needs to fight infection and heal. TPN can be given only through a CVC because otherwise the ingredients are too irritating to the veins.

Infection risks increase with TPN because it contains a lot of glucose (a type of sugar) to provide energy to your body's cells. Unfortunately, germs like to grow in conditions of high glucose and in malnourished patients who are very ill (typically, the type of patient who receives TPN). For all these reasons, strict sterile procedures for TPN lines must be followed.

12

Pressure Sores

Pressure sores (also known as bedsores) are epidemic among hospital and nursing home patients. If you're hospitalized for more than two weeks, the odds are about one in three that you'll get them.

And yet, according to the *New England Journal of Medicine*, almost all pressure sores can be prevented. If you're at risk for pressure sores, your advocate will have to play a big role in preventing them, by ensuring that your nurses are taking the proper steps to protect your skin. The best prevention: turning a bedridden patient every few hours.

Pressure sores are a problem only if your body stays in one position for too long. So patients who are severely ill or incapacitated are most at risk. Even if you're unable to get out of bed, you probably won't get pressure sores as long as you can reposition your body.

Pressure sores occur when the blood supply to areas of

the skin and underlying tissue is cut off. The tissue begins to die, leaving a large, open wound. They're more likely to occur in patients with poor circulation—for example, from heart disease or diabetes.

It doesn't take much pressure to stop the blood flow to skin and underlying tissues—you can make your skin blanch simply by pressing on it lightly with your thumb. The weight of the body against a mattress or wheelchair is more than enough to cut off the circulation to the skin. The critical factor in the formation of pressure sores isn't how much pressure is applied, but how long it lasts.

Through constant motion, most people unconsciously shift the pressure points on their bodies—while they sleep as well as when they're awake—so that circulation to any particular area isn't interrupted for more than a few minutes. In people who are immobile, constant pressure on a single area cuts off the circulation for so long that the skin and muscle begin to die. Pressure sores often form over a bony prominence—a hip or shoulder blade, for example—that presses into the mattress. Similarly, a person in a wheelchair may develop a pressure sore where the heel sits against the footrest.

We often think of pressure sores among patients who are chronically ill, but you're at risk even for shorter hospital stays. They can form quickly—within a couple of days in some cases.

Because pressure sores are more likely to occur in patients who are too ill to move, you'll have to count on your advocate to take the lead; he or she has a big role in preventing them.

Strategies to Prevent Pressure Sores

Traditionally, methods for preventing and treating pressure sores have been high-touch rather than high-tech. Frequent turning of the patient to relieve pressure on the skin is the mainstay of nursing care for pressure sores. The standard practice is to turn at-risk patients at least once every two hours.

Before going into the hospital, make a point of finding out what it does to prevent pressure sores. Studies show that a formal educational program for the nursing staff, and the use of specially trained teams, helps reduce the risk of pressure sores. In one nursing home, for example, the incidence of pressure sores dropped from 15 to 9 percent when a team was established; in a hospital, the incidence dropped from 20 percent to zero. Two other hospitals that began staff-education programs reduced the number of pressure sore cases by two-thirds and three-quarters, respectively.

The family can play a big role in preventing bedsores, by moving your limbs and massaging areas of your skin that are prone to breakdown. I remember a patient, Ethyl, who was admitted to the ICU with pneumonia.

Ethyl was in her eighties and bedridden in a fetal position. Her arms and legs couldn't be straightened at all, and she couldn't feed herself, clean herself, or move on her own. She was unable to speak but was able to hear very well. Ethyl's daughter had cared for her at home for the past eight years, and there was not a trace of a pressure sore or redness on her frail skin.

After only four days in the hospital, Ethyl's skin was breaking down on her hips and ankles. After eight years with not so much as a scratch on her skin, she now had pressure sores. I remember how upset her daughter was at seeing all her hard work erased in a few days.

There was a lesson for all of us in Ethyl's plight. It's easy to think that pressure sores are inevitable in certain patients. Yet we saw that they can be prevented even in a patient as old, frail, and ill as Ethyl. Her daughter had no special knowledge or expertise in preventing bedsores. She did have patience, persistence, and love.

Nutrition. Many bedridden patients suffer from malnutrition, which contributes to the formation of pressure sores. A study published in *Lancet*, the leading medical journal in Britain, found that giving patients vitamin C supplements (500 milligrams twice a day) reduces the size of pressure sores by 84 percent. You or your advocate can talk to your doctor or nurse about getting vitamin C supplements.

Mucopolysaccharide sulfate. One theory holds that clotting in the small blood vessels of the skin contributes to pressure sores. Mucopolysaccharide sulfate, an ointment that helps dissolve clots, has been shown to promote healing when applied twice daily to the affected skin in the early stages.

Measures for High-Risk Patients

In most cases, turning does a good job of preventing pressure sores, as long as it's done diligently. But if you're at special risk—for example, if you have poor circulation— or if you've already begun to develop pressure sores, ask your doctor and nurse about using a special mattress or bed.

A variety of designs have been used to attempt to prevent pressure sores and promote their healing. Some are designed to distribute pressure more evenly; others are intended to move the pressure points around.

Fluidized beds are filled with microscopic glass beads; they literally float the patient on a cushion of air. The beads circulate constantly in a stream of air, evenly distributing the weight of the body.

One study found that fluidized beds were five times more effective than standard therapy (that is, turning) at preventing pressure sores. Air-fluidized beds aren't widely used in hospitals and nursing homes. They're expensive and often impractical, because you can't elevate the head or foot of the bed. But if you're at high risk for getting pressure sores, you or your advocate can ask your doctor whether it's an option.

They may also be an option to help promote healing in patients who've already developed pressure sores. But even with them, it's harder to heal pressure sore than prevent them. One study of air-fluidized beds showed that only 14 percent of patients healed completely, and the average time required for healing was 119 days.

Low-air-loss beds work like air-fluidized beds, using air pressure to support the body. They haven't been studied as extensively, though. They consist of a regular hospital bed frame with a special large cushion through which air is constantly pumped. Their advantage over air-fluidized beds is that the head of the bed can be raised and lowered. Some of the beds also reposition patients automatically.

Alternating air mattresses look like ordinary air mattresses. A pump alternately inflates and deflates each air tube in the mattress, varying the pressure on the skin. Research indicates that the diameter of the individual air tubes in the mattress is important; 3-inch tubes are ineffective; 6-inch tubes are effective; and a double layer of 6-inch tubes is best of all. In one study, this last configuration reduced the incidence of pressure sores from 39 percent to 16 percent.

What Doesn't Work

Though widely used, eggcrate foam mattresses (foam mattresses shaped like eggcrates) and sheepskin pads don't relieve enough pressure to prevent pressure sores, according to the *New England Journal of Medicine*. Even worse is the doughnut cushion, an inflatable cushion that looks like a child's inner tube float. It actually *worsens* blood flow within the center of the ring. Contradicting the practice of many hospitals and nursing homes, the *New England Journal* says that it should not be used in the treatment of pressure sores.

13

Malnutrition

Malnutrition is a much bigger problem in hospitals than most people realize.

All too often, nurses, doctors and patients assume that weight loss is inevitable during a hospital stay, or even that it's a good thing.

It's not. Even if you have a few (or many) pounds you'd like to lose, a hospital stay is the worst possible time to go on a diet. Your body needs all the resources it can get to fight disease and infection.

It's been estimated that half of all patients don't get adequate nutrition while they're in the hospital. For example, a French study of elderly hospital patients found that 30 percent of men and 41 percent of women suffered from malnutrition during the first fifteen days of a hospital stay.

The study also found that *patients who lost weight had a greater risk of dying in the hospital.* A study from the United States found a similar relationship between malnutrition and death in the hospital or within three months of discharge.

The effects of malnutrition often masquerade as other problems. For example, lack of protein can slow or prevent healing of surgical wounds or pressure sores. Poor nutrition also weakens the immune system, preventing you from overcoming infections and leaving you susceptible to new ones.

Plenty of Food, but Who's Eating?

Ironically, there's no lack of food in hospitals. They have entire departments devoted to nutrition, and throughout the day the halls are full of carts carrying meals to patients—not necessarily good-tasting food, but plentiful nonetheless.

The problem in hospitals isn't lack of *food.* It's lack of *nutrition.* Many patients are starving despite the abundance, for a number of reasons.

- Many come into the hospital already malnourished as a result of their disease.
- In the hospital, their disease may leave them with little appetite. Many of those meals that go out to patients' rooms come back virtually untouched.
- There's little in the hospital environment to stimulate a good appetite. For example, there isn't much opportunity to exercise, and your regular schedule is disrupted.
- The food itself is often bland and overcooked. Special diets (such as salt-restricted diets) may compound the problem.

- Sometimes the disease itself interferes with your body's ability to take in and absorb nutrients.
- Sometimes disease or medications will alter your sense of taste, making food suddenly taste terrible.
- The body requires more, and different, nutrients when it's fighting disease or recovering from surgery or other diseases.

Protein and Calories Are Key

A traditional "balanced" diet may not be the best option when you're in the hospital. Your body has a higher need for protein and calories.

The body uses protein to rebuild tissues (for example, when wounds and surgical incisions are healing). Calories give you energy. (Unless you're on a restricted diet, the hospital is one place you shouldn't worry about getting too many calories!)

If your appetite is poor, ask your doctor or nurses whether family members can bring you high-protein and high-calorie foods and snacks from home. (Make sure the nurses know what you're eating so they can keep accurate records of your food intake.) Avoid foods that are fatty and/or high in sodium. Include fruits and vegetables, especially those high in vitamin C, which is required for tissue healing. Take vitamin supplements as well.

Perhaps most important, there's often not enough attention paid to your nutritional needs and whether they're being met. You may not have the strength or dexterity to feed yourself. You may be disoriented. You may have to get someone to help you eat, and this can take time. Try to have family or friends with you at mealtimes if you have trouble feeding yourself.

Knowing Whether You're Malnourished

Most hospitals have nutrition teams. If you're at risk for malnourishment, ask whether they can evaluate you.

A critical measure for nutrition is your albumin level. Albumin is protein that's dissolved in your blood, and it shows how much nourishment is actually getting to your body's tissues. (You can be malnourished even if you're eating a lot of food, if it isn't being absorbed into your bloodstream.) If you're at risk of malnutrition, your albumin levels should be checked with a blood test. These levels have proved to be good predictors of how well you'll recover. In one study, patients with low albumin levels (less than 34 grams per liter) were more likely to die, had longer hospital stays, and were readmitted sooner and more frequently than patients with normal albumin levels.

Strategies for Preventing Malnutrition

The first defense against malnutrition is to make sure that your nurses and doctors are paying attention to the problem. An astonishing amount of malnutrition can be avoided.

If you've lost weight recently, be sure your nutrition is reviewed when you go into the hospital. A study in one hospital found that only 42 percent of patients who were malnourished when admitted received any nutritional supplements.

Your body needs extra calories and protein to heal. If you're not taking in enough to meet your needs, your body "borrows" protein from other tissues to use in the healing process. That means it's fighting a battle on two fronts—against the disease and against itself. And when you're in the hospital, it's extremely difficult for your body to make up for the losses.

You may be too debilitated to ask or complain about hunger and weakness. You may not have any appetite. In these situations, your family and advocate play a critical role in ensuring that you get enough nutrition. Discuss this issue before you go into the hospital.

Watch Out for NPO Orders

If you're malnourished when you're admitted to the hospital, your condition can worsen if you have to fast for certain tests. If your doctors give NPO orders (that means, "nothing by mouth"), ask how you will receive nourishment—for example, by IV fluids, total parenteral nutrition (TPN, a special IV mixture that gives your body all the nutrients it needs to heal), a feeding tube placed into your stomach through your nose, or an incision into the abdomen.

If you need to have TPN or a feeding tube, you're at greater risk for infection (see page 141). The feeding tube can also irritate your skin or nasal passages, especially if it's left in for a while. Very soft and flexible tubes are available that don't cause pain or damage your skin; be sure to ask for one of these.

These procedures may cause you some discomfort, but remember: You need nutrition to heal, and this may be the only way to get it.

NPO orders should be in effect only as long as absolutely necessary.

If you're having a number of tests or procedures that require a fast, ask whether they can be scheduled close to one another so that you don't have to fast more than once.

Ask whether a modified diet is possible rather than a complete ban on foods—for example, clear liquids or a full liquid diet.

Treatment: Every Day Counts

Studies show that early intervention is critical for combating malnutrition. The longer you wait, the more your body has to make up.

If you're at all at risk for malnutrition, there seems to be little reason *not* to start giving you nutritional supplements as soon as you're admitted. They're unlikely to do you any harm, and getting them sooner rather than later can shorten your hospital stay. One study found that malnourished hospital patients who were started on some type of nutritional supplementation in the first three days of hospitalization had hospital stays that averaged three days shorter than patients whose supplements started on the fourth day or later.

In fact, if you know you'll be going into the hospital, you can start giving yourself supplements at home. Check with your doctor first, however. You can buy them at your grocery store or your local pharmacy without a prescription. Don't confuse them with vitamin or herbal "supplements"—you need a *nutritional* supplement. The most common brand is Ensure. If you're not sure what to get, ask your pharmacist.

14

Complications of Surgery

Surgery is safer than ever. Newer techniques, such as laparoscopic surgery, are faster and require smaller incisions, resulting in less trauma to your body and shorter recovery times. New technologies allow surgeons to operate on even the finest structures in the body, using devices that let them work at a microscopic level. Better imaging gives surgeons a more accurate picture of what's going on in your body beforehand, so they encounter fewer surprises when they go in.

But surgery has its own unique risks, in addition to those for any hospital stay. Besides the things that can go wrong with the operation itself, you can suffer from side effects of anesthesia, infection, and respiratory problems.

Also, surgery—especially major surgery—tends to be a more aggressive solution than nonsurgical alternatives and can be harder to "undo" if problems arise. If you take a drug and experience undesirable side effects, your doctor can discontinue the drugs and often the side effects will go away. With surgery, you either have to live with the results or, perhaps, face a second operation to fix the problem.

Questions to Ask About Your Surgery

Here are some questions to ask your surgeon or primary-care physician before you have an operation.

Are There Alternatives to Surgery?

Sometimes, surgery isn't the only answer to a medical problem. Medicines or other nonsurgical treatments, such as a change in diet or special exercises, might help you just as well or more. Ask your surgeon or primary-care doctor about the benefits and risks of these other choices.

One alternative may be *watchful waiting,* in which your doctor and you check to see if your problem gets worse or better. If it gets worse, you may need surgery right away. If it gets better, you may be able to postpone surgery, perhaps indefinitely.

If you have an inflamed appendix or gallbladder, of course, you don't have to think very long or hard about whether to have an operation. But often the picture is less clear.

For example, Peter was recovering from a gunshot wound. The bullet was lodged near Peter's spine. The original surgeon left the bullet in place to avoid damaging the nerve. Later, the bone surrounding the spinal cord became infected.

Peter saw two specialists—a surgeon and an internist. After reviewing a set of X rays, the surgeon recommended an immediate operation to remove the bullet and treat the bone infection. Without the operation, he said, the bone would continue to degenerate and Peter could expect long-term pain and disability.

The internist, however, reviewed the same X rays and came up with exactly the opposite conclusion: The infection was getting better on its own, and the bullet was out of harm's way. Surgery would be risky and could interfere with the healing process. The best thing to do, he said, was to leave it be.

Peter didn't have the surgery, and eventually his spine healed on its own.

That example underscores something to keep in mind when you're talking to a surgeon: We're all more comfortable with what we know. Internists, who don't perform surgery, often lean toward nonsurgical solutions, such as drugs or physical therapy. Surgeons, not surprisingly, tend to favor surgical solutions. As the old saying goes, "To a man with a hammer, everything looks like a nail."

That's not to say that either side is necessarily right or wrong, or that a surgeon will always recommend surgery. It simply means you need to be aware of how the doctor's background may influence his or her advice.

What Type of Surgery Should I Have?

There may be more than one type of operation for your condition. Be sure you know all of the surgical options. Find out *exactly* what operation the surgeon is recommending. Ask whether other types of procedures could be used to treat your condition, and why the surgeon is recommending this particular procedure.

Newer techniques may be less traumatic, less painful, and faster to heal than traditional operations. For example, laparascopic surgery uses a viewing scope and tools that are inserted through small incisions, often small enough to require only a Band-Aid after the operation is over. However, these newer techniques require different skills. If a surgeon hasn't been trained in newer techniques, he or she may not be able to give you up-to-date information. It pays to investigate. Get a second opinion, or do some research on your own.

What Are the Benefits of Having the Operation?

Ask your surgeon what you will gain by having the operation. For example, a hip replacement may allow you to walk again easily without pain.

Ask how long the benefits are likely to last. For some procedures, it is not unusual for the benefits to last for only a short time. You might need a second operation at a later date. For other procedures, the benefits may last a lifetime.

When finding out about the benefits of the operation, be realistic. Sometimes patients expect too much and are disappointed with the outcome, or results. Ask your doctor if there is any published information about the outcomes of the procedure.

Find out the track record of success for the type of operation you're supposed to get. Some operations, despite their popularity, aren't all that effective. For example, recent studies suggest that patients who undergo surgery for back pain are no more likely to find relief than patients who are treated nonsurgically. Similarly, studies of arthroscopic knee surgery found that it's often ineffective.

And be sure you understand the operation's *long-term* effectiveness. Some operations provide a permanent cure; others don't. Knee and hip replacements, for example, typically last about ten to fifteen years before they wear out. That's not to say these operations aren't worthwhile—but when you're weighing benefits and risks, it's important to understand exactly what kind of benefit you can expect.

What Are the Risks of Having the Operation?

All operations carry some risk. You need to weigh the benefits of the operation against the risks of complications or side effects.

Complications are unplanned events, such as infection, too much bleeding, reaction to anesthesia, accidental injury or respiratory distress.

In addition, you may experience *side effects* after the operation. For the most part, side effects can be anticipated. For example, your surgeon knows that there will be swelling and some soreness at the site of the operation.

What Kind of Anesthesia Will I Need?

Your surgeon can tell you whether the operation calls for local, regional, or general anesthesia, and why this form of anesthesia is recommended for your procedure. *Local anesthesia* numbs only a part of your body for a short period of time—for example, a tooth and the surrounding gum. Not all procedures done with local anesthesia are painless, however. *Regional anesthesia* numbs a larger portion of your body—for example, the lower part of your body—for a few hours. In most cases, you will be awake with regional anesthesia. *General anesthesia* numbs your entire body for the entire time of the surgery. You will be unconscious if you have general anesthesia. Usually the type of operation dictates the type of anesthesia used.

Anesthesia is quite safe for most patients and is usually administered by a specialized physician (anesthesiologist) or nurse anesthetist. Both are highly skilled and have been specially trained to give anesthesia. However, it is important to tell the anesthesiologist your smoking history or any other respiratory conditions.

How Long Will It Take Me to Recover?

Your surgeon can tell you how you might feel and what you will be able to do or not do the first few days, weeks, or months after surgery. Ask how long you will be in the hospital. Find out what kind of supplies, equipment, and any other help you will need when you go home. Knowing what to expect can help you cope better with recovery.

Ask when you can start regular exercise again and go back to work. Also ask about any limitations on your activities, so you don't do anything to slow the recovery process. Lifting a ten-pound bag of potatoes may not seem like a big deal a week after your operation, but it could be.

Where Will the Operation Be Done?

Most surgeons practice at one or two local hospitals. Find out where your operation will be performed. Have many operations like yours been done in this hospital? Some operations have higher success rates at hospitals that do many of those procedures. Ask your doctor about the success rate at the hospital he or she plans to send you to. If the hospital has a low success rate for the operation in question, you can ask to have the operation at another hospital.

Today, many operations are done in a doctor's office, a special surgical center, or a day surgery unit of a hospital. Outpatient surgery is often a good choice, depending on the type of operation and your condition. As we've seen, the less time spent in the hospital, the fewer opportunities for something to go wrong. You may be safer recovering at home.

The key issue to consider for outpatient surgery is how your recovery will go after the procedure. Consider whether you'll be able to take care of yourself when you arrive home. If not, do you have someone to assist you during convalescence? You will also need someone to drive you home if a procedure involves general anesthesia or results in physical impairment such as a cast, stitches, or pain.

If complications occur, what are your options for being admitted to a hospital for more extended care? Many centers are freestanding, meaning they are not connected to a hospital. Medical and nursing care may not be as readily available. Discuss these issues with your physician and know what options are available if things don't go according to the original plan. Be wary of the answers such as, "Don't worry, everything will be fine," or "You won't need to be admitted to the hospital." Get a *specific* answer. If you can't get one from your doctor, get a second opinion. Surprises can happen.

For example, David had a hernia repaired as an outpatient. He felt fine after he woke up from surgery, was able to eat and drink, and his pain was controlled, so he was discharged home.

But Loretta had a different experience when she had her gallbladder removed as an outpatient. After the anesthesia was supposed to wear off, she was still feeling groggy. Her blood pressure was low and she was vomiting. As the day wore on, Loretta didn't improve, despite receiving medications to stop vomiting. It was apparent that Loretta couldn't go home in this condition. She was admitted to the hospital, where an IV line was inserted to replace the fluids she'd lost from vomiting. The next morning Loretta was fine and ready to go home.

Find out what kinds of procedures the center is qualified to do. You can call your local hospital or ambulatory surgical center to ask for a list of approved procedures that can be done as outpatient. Review boards give guidelines for approval of the center and license them to do procedures. They may impose restrictions on which procedures can be performed as outpatient. The center should be able to tell you.

If your doctor recommends inpatient surgery for a procedure that is usually done as outpatient surgery, or vice versa, ask why.

Don't forget to check with your insurance companies

before any procedure to be sure it's covered. Also be sure the insurance company isn't pushing you to have outpatient surgery when you really should be an inpatient receiving extended care. Call your doctor's office if you encounter problems with insurance coverage. Often the office can send a letter to the insurance company requesting a change in the coverage due to your specific condition.

CHECKING OUT AMBULATORY SURGERY CENTERS

If you're having surgery in an ambulatory surgery center (sometimes called a "day surgery" center), call your health plan or visit the center to find out:

- If your health plan will cover your care there.
- If it is licensed. Then check to see if it is accredited by a group such as the Joint Commission on Accreditation of Healthcare Organizations (telephone 630-792-5800; Web site http://www.jcaho.org) or the Accreditation Association for Ambulatory Healthcare (847-676-9610). The accreditation certificate should be posted in the facility.
- If it is approved for the procedure you're having.
- How well trained and experienced the center's health care professionals are.
- Whether the center is affiliated with a hospital. If it is not, find out how the center will handle any emergency that could happen during your visit.

Getting a Second Opinion

Second opinions can save lives. Rebecca was admitted to the hospital with chest pain. She was thirty-four years old and athletic, and her initial lab tests and electrocardiogram (EKG) were normal. So her physician was sure that whatever was wrong with her, it wasn't her heart.

During Rebecca's hospital stay, she began to have more episodes of chest pain. But her EKG and blood pressure were always normal. Prescribed treatments didn't help. Rebecca felt awful, and nothing was helping. She and her family felt helpless.

I told Rebecca and the family that if they were dissatisfied with the medical care, they should ask for a second opinion. They had no idea that they could do so. A second physician concluded that she did have heart disease after all. Rebecca received the right treatment for her blocked heart vessels and began to improve. Without the second opinion, she could have suffered a crippling heart attack.

Insurance companies may not always pay for consultations outside their plan, but it is important to consider the potential benefits of another opinion, even if you have to pay for it yourself.

It's surprising how many people don't realize they can ask for the second opinion. Patients have told me they can't ask for another opinion for fear of making the physician angry or hurting his or her feelings, or that "the doctor knows what's best." I've also heard patients say things like, "I have to trust her judgment," or "This doctor is the only one in town so his opinion must be correct," or "The hospital wouldn't hire a bad doctor," or

"She has been our family doctor for years, so she knows what I need."

A second opinion isn't about whether you trust your doctor. It's simply a matter of two heads being better than one. Much of medicine comes down to judgment calls, and another doctor may look at your problem in a different light.

And speaking of other opinions, I counsel patients to consider their *own* opinion as well. Don't ignore your own doubts and common sense. Trust your instincts; you may not have a medical degree, but you know your own body better than anyone else.

It is also surprising that many nurses don't know that patients can get a second opinion—even if they're already in the hospital. One of the first things we learn in nursing school is the patient's right to choose and refuse. But often nurses keep quiet because they don't want to be labeled as troublemakers, overstep their bounds, or contradict the doctor.

Ideally, the second opinion will agree with the first. If it doesn't, however, keep in mind that second opinions aren't infallible, either. Often there isn't a "right" answer, just a variety of informed opinions. But getting two opinions is like shining two lights on the problem. You can see it more clearly.

If you're still unsure, you can seek more opinions, or get more information to try to resolve the differences. Or you may choose to go with your original doctor's recommendation. Even in that case, however, the second opinion helps you and the doctor be sure you've covered all the possibilities and have arrived at the best decision.

RISK ALERT

If you get a second opinion, make sure to get your records from the first doctor so that the second doctor doesn't have to repeat tests.

Strategies to Reduce Surgical Risk

As soon you learn that you'll need an operation, there are steps you can take to reduce the risk of complications.

Try to Stay Healthy

Try to have your operation while you're still healthy.

Surgery is a big step, and it's natural to want to put it off as long as possible. But once you've decided to have the operation, it's usually in your interest to have it sooner rather than later, before your condition worsens. The healthier you are overall, the better the chances that you'll avoid complications during or after the operation.

Sometimes weeks or even months can be lost simply trying to get an appointment to see the doctor. For elective surgery, you'll probably need at least one office visit with the surgeon before your operation is scheduled. You may need to have additional tests conducted as well. Your best bet is to make these appointments as soon as you can, even if you're not yet 100 percent sure about having the operation. You can always change your mind later if you need to—right up until the time they put you under anesthesia.

If you're diabetic, be sure your glucose levels are under control, to prevent hyperglycemia during the operation.

Know What's Involved

Before you have an operation, the surgeon will obtain your *informed consent*. (The anesthesiologist will also obtain a separate informed consent from you.) This discussion may take place in the hospital or before you go in. Ideally, the sooner you have the discussion the better. But sometimes the doctor has to wait for test results to figure out what's going on—so the informed-consent discussion might take place just before the procedure.

Consider having your advocate or another family member present to ask any questions you may not think of, and to help you remember later what was discussed. It's also a good idea to take notes.

Informed consent is a concept that emerged from legal cases. From a legal standpoint, a surgeon can't operate on you without your consent (except in an emergency where you're unable to give consent). But the courts recognized that for complex medical procedures, consent doesn't mean much unless you truly understand what you're agreeing to.

To give informed consent, you must be told:

- who will perform the operation
- the nature of the operation
- the chances of success

- the risks of complications
- other alternatives you could choose, along with their chances of success and risks
- the likely consequences of not having the procedure

You can learn a lot from how the surgeon handles informed consent. Does he or she regard it as a legal formality to be gotten out of the way as quickly as possible, or an opportunity to address any concerns you have?

Don't sign the consent forms until you feel that all of your questions have been answered. Every operation involves some degree of risk. Be sure you understand what those risks are—and that you are sure you're willing to take them.

If you have any lingering questions or concerns, get them answered before proceeding with the surgery. Even if you are in the operating room, you can ask questions and ask to speak to your doctor before beginning surgery.

Discuss Anesthesia and Pain Management

Also talk with the surgeon and/or the anesthesiologist about what type of pain management will be available after surgery, and the benefits and side effects of each method. Some pain may be unavoidable, but keep in mind that you won't get a medal for toughing it out after an operation. Your body will heal faster if your pain is controlled.

Find out who will actually be administering the anesthesia. Will the anesthesiologist *personally* monitor you through the entire operation, or will someone else, such as a resident, be doing it under the anesthesiologist's supervision? There's not necessarily anything wrong with that arrangement; it depends on what you're comfortable with.

If others will be involved, will the anesthesiologist be present in the operating room during your entire procedure? You have the right to insist on these things, but you have to ask to make sure. Make sure it's all spelled out in the informed consent form before you sign it. Write it in by hand if you need to.

Know your medical history, and be sure the anesthesiologist knows it too. Have you ever had general anesthesia before? How did you react to it? Does the anesthesiologist have access to your medical records from previous operations? Has he or she reviewed them?

Eat and Drink

Be sure to increase your water intake, especially a few days before surgery. Older people, especially, are frequently dehydrated. You may be dehydrated even if you don't feel thirsty.

Poor nutrition delays recovery and puts you at greater risk of complications (see Chapter 13). Be sure to eat well-balanced meals that include plenty of protein and vitamins.

Don't Smoke

Smokers heal more slowly and have a much higher risk of surgical complications. It causes the blood vessels to constrict, decreasing blood flow to tissues and interfering with healing. Smoking also increases the risk of lung complications after surgery. If you smoke, you're also at a higher risk of developing blood clots.

To avoid these problems, it's best to give up smoking altogether before your operation. Simply cutting back isn't enough to prevent the complications. If you can't quit, at the very least don't smoke within twelve hours of your operation, and try not to smoke afterward.

Arrange Your Aftercare

Make sure you've made all the arrangements you need for after your operation. You may need assistance at home for a few days or weeks.

If you're having outpatient surgery, be sure to have some one available to drive you home when it's done. You will be sedated and won't be able to drive. If you'll be staying in the hospital, you may not be able to drive after you're discharged, especially if you're taking pain medication.

Fast the Night Before

You will probably be given instructions about not eating the night before your surgery. Be sure you follow them. This is a hard rule to follow because of hunger and thirst, but it will help prevent complications while you're under anesthesia. Otherwise, food or liquids can be vomited up and get lodged in your lungs, causing a severe form of pneumonia.

In the Hospital

Once you've been admitted to the hospital, it's a good idea to review your care with your nurses and doctors. Ask your nurses to explain what will happen to you. You may have heard much of this already from the doctor, but nurses may have a different perspective. The more points of view you have, the better your understanding of what to expect. And it's a good way to make sure all your caregivers are on the same wavelength.

Take Steps to Prevent Infections

We've discussed infections elsewhere, but there are some special considerations to keep in mind for surgical infections. An operation puts you at high risk for infection, because it breaks through your body's most effective defense against germs: your skin. The incision creates a pathway for germs to invade, so good postoperative care is designed to keep them at bay until your wound heals, and to help it heal as quickly as possible.

The Centers for Disease Control convened a panel of experts to create a set of guidelines to help prevent post-surgical infections. While most of these guidelines are directed at surgeons and operating-room personnel, several are relevant for patients as well.

If you have an active infection—even one as minor as a head cold—it's better to postpone the surgery until the infection clears up, if possible. Your doctor will have to weigh the risks of infection against the risk of putting off the operation. The CDC guidelines note that mupirocin ointment, applied inside the nasal passages, kills *Staphylococcus aureus,* a type of bacterium that's often responsible for surgical infections. Staph bacteria often colonize the nose, producing no symptoms, and can spread by way of the hands to surgical wounds. Studies suggest that mupirocin, applied before surgery, reduces the risk of postsurgical infection.

The CDC panel also recommends that hair *not* be removed from the surgical site unless it will interfere with the operation. Traditionally, hair is removed before an operation. Shaving the site the night before increases your risk of infection, as it creates microscopic breaks in the skin where germs can grow. Shaving or clipping the site immediately before the operation is less likely to cause infection than if it's done the night before. Depilatories, or no hair removal, are associated with a much lower infection rate. Depilatories, however, can irritate the skin, so some experts recommend not removing the hair from the site unless it's absolutely necessary.

Ask your doctor whether you'll be given antimicrobial prophylaxis (AMP). You receive a dose of antibiotics to help control any microbes that make their way into the surgical site during the operation. You receive the drugs intravenously, beginning just before the operation and continuing for a few hours after the incision is closed. It's not used for all types of surgery—for example, it doesn't help if the wound is already infected—but it may be appropriate for you.

Make Sure the Surgical Site Is Marked

Don't assume that your surgical team knows what part of you they're operating on and why. Surgeons perform a lot of operations, and while mixups are rare, they do happen.

For example, Gloria had a skin tag—a flap of excess skin—on her rectum that was causing a lot of problems. It was large and inflamed most of the time. Finally, she got up her courage and decided to get it removed.

When Gloria came out of surgery, she had a lot of pain and a dressing packing in her rectum. When she asked how the operation went, she was told that the hemorrhoids had come out just fine. Gloria asked, "What about the skin tag?"

The surgeon had removed her hemorrhoids—a procedure she hadn't asked for and probably didn't need—and hadn't removed the skin tag. Luckily, in the long run, she probably didn't suffer any permanent damage. But she did experience a lot of discomfort for a procedure she didn't need. And she still needed to have the skin tag removed.

Sometimes the consequences can be more severe. A surgeon may operate on the wrong body part. Or get the part right but do the wrong procedure. Or get the part and the procedure right but have the wrong patient.

One simple step can go a long way toward preventing mixups. When you meet with your surgeon before the operation, show the site and have him or her mark it with an indelible marker. The healthy side can also be marked with a "No." That's especially important when the surgeon is operating on something that comes in pairs—knees, breasts, kidneys, lungs.

If you meet with others on the team—such as the anesthesiologist, operating room nurse, or technician—show them the correct site as well. The more people who know, the less likely that a mistake will go unnoticed.

The Joint Commission on Accreditation of Healthcare

Organizations has identified a number of risk factors for wrong-site surgery. Your risk is increased if:

- more than one surgeon is involved in the case, either because multiple procedures are needed or because the case was transferred from one surgeon to another (for example, one with specialized expertise)
- you're scheduled to undergo more than one procedure during a single trip to the operating room, especially if the procedures are on opposite sides of your body
- the surgical team is in a hurry, especially if the operation is scheduled for an unusual time or if there's pressure to speed up preoperative procedures
- you have a physical condition, such as obesity, that requires special setup or positioning

Discuss Allergies

Know your allergies and be sure your doctor, the nurses, and the person giving you the anesthetic all know if you have allergies. You could have an allergic reaction to the anesthesia.

Don't assume that you're allergy-free just because you've never had a reaction in the past. You can develop an allergic reaction to any substance at any time. If you feel strange after receiving a medicine, tell the nurse immediately. Medicines are available to stop the allergic reaction (see also Chapter 10).

Heading Off Wound Infections

Earlier, we discussed ways to avoid infections. Those precautions are even more important after you've had a major operation. After all, if an IV line or urinary catheter provides a path for germs to enter your body, a surgical incision is like a six-lane superhighway. *Absolutely nobody should touch the area around your incision without washing their hands and taking steps to avoid contaminating the site.* (That includes you, by the way.) To avoid wound infections, follow the recommendations in Chapter 11.

Even with these precautions, wound infections can still take hold. So the second thing you can do to protect yourself is to watch for early signs of infection and tell your nurses if they appear.

Signs of infection include abnormal redness or swelling at the incision site, pus or foul-smelling discharge, or unusual pain or tenderness. The site may feel warm. You'll need to be extra vigilant, because these signs can be masked by the ordinary process of healing. After all, surgical incisions are likely to be tender and oozy.

Your nurses will be watching the site for signs of infection, and they're trained to know the difference between what's normal and what isn't. But you can help them catch infections early by paying attention to what your body is telling you. Are you experiencing more pain than you or the nurses expected? Do you feel early signs of fever—such as aching joints, chills, or sweats? Do you feel dizzy or disoriented? Do you feel worse and weaker as your recovery progresses, instead of better and stronger? Let your nurses know. These can all be signs of infection, and the sooner you catch it, the easier it is to control.

Avoiding Lung Complications

Operations are hard on lungs. While you're under general anesthesia, a ventilator mechanically inflates and deflates them. Afterward, postsurgical pain makes it difficult to take the deep breaths that keep the lungs' airways open and clear. And lying flat on your back during the operation and recovery makes it hard for your lungs to clear out fluids. As a result, respiratory complications such as fluid buildup, pneumonia, atelectasis, and collapsed lung are possibilities. (Atelectasis is the result of lungs not expanding fully in the smaller airways. Pneumonia and respiratory failure can result.)

Exercise Your Lungs

After surgery (or with any prolonged bed rest), you must exercise your lungs to keep the airways open and free of extra fluid. To exercise your lungs, take in as deep a breath as you can. Suck in some more air in and hold it for a few seconds, then exhale fully and push out everything you have in your lungs. Repeat this exercise at least ten times. You may be given a little breathing tube called a spirometer to blow in and out of. Be sure to do the exercises as often as you are told, even if they hurt. Coughing at the end of the deep breaths will help clear your lungs of mucus that has gotten trapped.

Keep Moving!

Prolonged bed rest after surgery decreases your circulation. Muscles become weak and can waste away in a matter of hours.

Activity and leg exercises prevent blood clots from forming in the weak muscle tissue. Blood clots can travel through your body to any organ, including your lungs, brain, or heart, and result in serious complications or death.

Your nurses will tell you when you can get out of bed and will assist you so that you don't fall. It may be painful at first, but it's critical that you get on your feet as soon as you can. Walk if you're up to it; if not, at least sit up in a chair. Walk to the bathroom instead of using the bedpan or commode. (But be sure your nurses have told you it's okay to get out of bed, and ask for assistance if you need it. Otherwise, you could be at risk for falling. See Chapter 15.)

Exercise your legs to minimize the weakness: Raise your legs up and down five times. Bend your knee and straighten your leg five times. Stretch your toes down and up.

Watch for Signs of Pneumonia

These measures can go a long way toward preventing postsurgical pneumonia, but you're still at risk. Watch for early signs of pneumonia and be sure it's treated aggressively if it occurs (see pages 135–136).

15

Falls

Falls—in and out of the hospital—are the second leading cause of accidental death in the United States, after auto accidents. Especially for older patients, falls can be catastrophic: About half of those who suffer serious fall injuries never recover normal function. The most common injury is a hip fracture. A study of hospital falls by the Iowa Hospital Association found that 69 percent occurred in the patient's room and 15 percent in the bathroom.

When Are You Most at Risk?

The Joint Commission on Accreditation of Healthcare Organizations, the organization that accredits hospitals, found a number of risk factors related to fatal falls:

- Altered mental status, due to chronic mental illness or drug effects.
- A history of prior falls.
- Sedation.
- The use of anticoagulants (that is, blood-thinning medications); these drugs promote bleeding and so worsen the effects of falling.
- Recent environmental changes—for example, a transfer to a new room.
- Having to use the bathroom. Many patients who are supposed to be restricted to bed don't wait for the nurse's help and try to get out of bed themselves.
- Nights, weekends, and holidays. Falls are more likely to occur during off-hour shifts.
- Malfunction or misuse of bed alarms (sometimes the alarms are intentionally disabled because they go off when patients are simply moving around in bed).

Strategies to Avoid Falls

Patients are often surprised when they fall. You can use the JCAHO list to know when you need to exercise extra caution, but it's also useful to follow common-sense guidelines.

Don't Get Up Without Help

The best way to avoid falls is to follow one simple rule: *Don't try to get into or out of your bed without assistance.*

Even in the best of circumstances, hospital beds are tricky to negotiate. They can be raised and lowered, meaning you might have a bigger step down to the floor than you expect. And it's easy to trip over the paraphernalia surrounding the bed. You can trip over IV or catheter lines. You can stumble against IV poles or other equipment. A bed tray may roll away from you unexpectedly if you grab onto it for support.

When you are getting into or out of bed, you can use the bed rails for support, but don't climb *over* a bed rail. Ask the nurse to lower it. Many hospital beds have half rails, so they can be raised around your head and shoulders to keep you from falling out of bed, and left down at the foot of the bed so you can more easily get in and out.

If you're having problems controlling your bladder or bowels, let your nurses know so they can respond quickly when you call for assistance. You may need a urinary catheter or Depends; unpleasant, perhaps, but far preferable to a broken hip or other fall-related injury. And if you have to go to the bathroom, ring for the nurse early and often. If you're at risk for falling, don't try to go to the bathroom by yourself—if worse comes to worse, it's better to have the kind of accident that a nurse can clean up rather than one that results in a broken hip or other injury.

Communicate with the Nursing Staff

The JCAHO study found that falls often result from poor communication among and with the nursing staff.

Good communication starts with an accurate assessment. You or your advocate can ask nurses whether they've assessed your risk of falling. (It should be a routine part of the nursing assessment.) If you *are* at risk, ask what measures they're taking to prevent falls. Make sure nurses on all shifts know about and are following these measures.

Whenever there's a change in scenery, you're at greater risk. If you have to be moved—for example, from one nursing unit to another, or from the hospital room to a rehab unit—make sure you know where the bathroom is and that the nurses on each shift know what measures they should be following.

Get the Right Equipment

If there's an alarm on your bed, make sure it works. The alarms are activated by weight and sound an alarm for the nurses if the bed is empty.

Not every bed has an alarm. They're most often used with patients who are disoriented or confused. A malfunctioning alarm is worse than no alarm at all, because it creates a false sense of security. The nurses will assume that if the alarm isn't sounding, everything is fine.

If you or your loved one is at risk for falling, see if a special low bed is available. That way, if you do fall, you're less likely to get injured. Otherwise, ask the nurses to keep the bed at its lowest position whenever possible.

Watch Where You Walk

Only about 5 percent of patient falls occur in the corridor or common areas of the hospital; most occur in the patient's room or bathrooom. However, you still need to be careful when you're walking. Most important: Be sure you have a good pair of nonslip footwear. Water and other fluids are often spilled on the floor in the hospital. Never walk in the hospital without proper footwear. You never know what you may step on!

Avoiding Other Hazards

Use caution and common sense wherever you're in the hospital. Hospital corridors are often crowded with unused beds, food carts, and other equipment. Hospital rooms have valves and racks that can give you a nasty bump on the head. Doctors and nurses may be rushing through the halls to deal with an emergency. Family members and visitors will be coming and going. Remember that you're in a public place, and take the same precautions as you would elsewhere.

16

Misdiagnosis

Misdiagnosis can harm you in two ways: You won't get treated properly for the problems you *do* have, and you're exposed to treatments—and their risks—for problems you *don't* have.

It's a dangerous misconception to assume that your diagnosis is clear and definite. That's simply not true. Studies consistently find that many hospitalized patients receive the wrong diagnosis. One recent study, for example, found a misdiagnosis rate of 20 percent in the ICU at Cleveland Clinic, one of the top hospitals in the nation. Almost half of those misdiagnoses were considered to be major because they led doctors to prescribe the wrong treatment. A study from Johns Hopkins Hospital found major diagnostic errors in 9.5 percent of cases.

In many cases, a diagnosis really represents an educated guess. Granted, the doctor is highly educated, and the guesses are usually very good ones. But for many disorders, the diagnosis is uncertain to some degree and should be considered that way. In other words, one should approach the diagnosis with something of an open mind. Even if the evidence points strongly in one direction today, new evidence may change the picture tomorrow.

Tests are important in arriving at or confirming a diagnosis, but they're not always definitive either. They can be done incorrectly, or the results can be misreported, but those cases are rare. More commonly, they produce a result that is ambiguous, is open to interpretation, or could support more than one diagnosis. That's where the doctor's judgment comes into play.

Misdiagnosis doesn't only mean finding the wrong illness. The doctor may figure out the right illness but misjudge its *severity*. That can lead to under- or overtreatment. For example, most cancers must be staged to determine how far they've spread in the patient's body. Treatments are very different, depending on the stage to which the cancer has progressed.

Warning Signs of Misdiagnosis

Here are some warning signs that you may have been misdiagnosed.

The Treatment Isn't Working the Way It Should

If you're not seeing the results that you and your doctor expected, it may be a sign that you're treating the wrong condition.

Treatment failures don't *always* mean you've been misdiagnosed; they can happen for any number of reasons. But if your doctor can't find any good reason that treatment failed—or if you've tried different treatments and they all come up short—it may be time to reexamine the diagnosis. Often a physician will counsel you to wait a little longer rather than reconsider the diagnosis. That may be good advice, but be sure you know what the potential risks might be from waiting. You also have the right to ask for a second opinion if you're not satisfied with the progress of your care.

The Doctor Is Defensive

A good doctor encourages your questions and respects your concerns. If the doctor gets defensive, seems to resent your inquiries, or dismisses them, it may be a sign that he or she isn't willing to consider other points of view. There are few absolutes in medicine, and a doctor who's overconfident or defensive may miss important clues if the diagnosis is in fact wrong.

Some doctors still subscribe to the idea that they can't show any signs of doubt in front of patients—that doing so will undermine their patients' trust and confidence in them. Other doctors simply don't like to be challenged—by patients, nurses, colleagues, or anyone else. Those attitudes can get in the way of effective diagnosis and treatment. Remember, you have the right to change your doctor if you don't like how you're being treated.

Test Results Seem Out of Whack

When researchers look back at cases of misdiagnosis, they often find obvious warning signs—including test results that clearly contradict the original diagnosis. Yet at the time, many of these signs were ignored or explained away. Why? It's simply human nature. Once we "know" a thing to be true, we all have a tendency to focus on evidence to support what we believe and ignore evidence that doesn't fit or contradicts it.

Therefore, it's not uncommon for doctors and others to explain away test results that don't fit the diagnosis they've already established. They may assume that the test was done incorrectly, or the results reported incorrectly, or simply that the results are thrown off for unknown reasons.

If you've had tests to confirm your diagnosis, ask your doctor to explain the results. Don't settle for a vague response like, "They're about what we expected." Find out whether all of the tests support the diagnosis. Ask if any of the results are anomalous or unexpected. If so, ask the doctor to explain why.

You Have a Feeling Things Aren't Right

Though you lack the doctor's medical expertise and training, you know your body best. Trust your instincts, and listen to what your body is trying to tell you. If you have any doubts, get another opinion, especially if you think something's wrong but the doctor says you're fine. It could be lifesaving. If you're still not sure, get a third opinion.

Don't worry about offending the doctor. A good doctor welcomes a second opinion, and admits to limitations of knowledge. If you wish, do some independent research (see Resources). Find out what tests are typically done to diagnose the condition. Were those tests done in your case? Do the reported symptoms seem to fit? But don't try to diagnose yourself. If you have concerns, take what you've learned and discuss it with your doctor.

RISK ALERT: TOO MUCH TREATMENT?

Diagnosis doesn't always lead directly to treatment. The fact that you've been diagnosed with a disease doesn't necessarily mean you need treatment, or at least not right away. Sometimes the better option is *watchful waiting*—keeping an eye on the situation and seeing what develops.

That's especially true when the risk of complications far outweigh the potential benefits of treatment. For example, Timothy, a seventy-six-year-old patient, was diagnosed with a bowel obstruction and was admitted to the hospital in critical condition. Timothy also had kidney disease and a heart condition. A bowel obstruction is life threatening and usually requires immediate surgery. But in this case, the risk of complications from general anesthesia were so high that the doctors chose to start with conservative measures and see what developed. They inserted a tube into Timothy's stomach to drain fluid and try to relieve pressure on the obstruction.

Over the next two weeks, Timothy suffered from one complication after another. But finally the obstruction began to clear and his condition improved. He avoided having an operation that he might not have survived.

Watchful waiting is almost always a judgment call and depends on the individual circumstances. Some doctors are more comfortable with the idea, while others tend to favor more aggressive action. And some pursue a more aggressive approach because they think that's what the patient wants. Don't assume that the most aggressive option is the best one. Talk to your doctor, and be sure you understand the benefits and risks of all your options. Remember, *you* have the last word on whether to choose or decline the treatments your doctor recommends.

Strategies to Reduce the Risk of Misdiagnosis

Ask Your Doctor!

So how can you, as a mere layperson, tell whether your doctor's diagnosis is accurate or definitive? Surprisingly, you can learn a lot simply by asking, "How certain are you that the diagnosis is correct?" Many patients assume that when the physician delivers a diagnosis, he or she is certain. If asked directly, however, most physicians will answer you honestly.

The doctor will probably be able to give you only a rough guess of how certain the diagnosis is. But it's still an important piece of information to have as your treatment progresses. Say, for example, that your treatment doesn't seem to be working. If your doctor is 95 percent sure that the diagnosis is correct, the next logical step is to try another treatment for the same condition. But if the doctor is only 65 percent certain, a treatment failure may be a sign to reconsider the diagnosis before proceeding with more treatments. Or if the recommended course of treatment is especially difficult or dangerous, you may want to insist on getting a clearer diagnosis before you go forward.

Here are some other questions to ask the doctor:

- How did you arrive at the diagnosis?
- What tests have been done to establish, confirm, or rule out the diagnosis?
- What additional tests, if any, will be done, and why?
- How definitive are the tests? What do they rule out? What *don't* they rule out?
- How accurate are the tests? How often do they result in false-positives (that is, they falsely indicate that you have the condition when you really don't)? How often do they result in false-negatives (that is, they indicate you don't have the condition when you really do)?
- Should the tests be repeated to confirm the diagnosis? Should other tests be performed? If so, what are they?
- What other diseases or conditions produce similar symp-

toms and/or test results? How do you rule out one or the other?

- Do you (that is, the doctor) plan to consult another physician to review the diagnosis? If so, can this be done *before* you (the patient) go into the hospital?

Be Alert for Imaging Errors

The most common type of misdiagnosis involves radiology and other types of medical imaging, such as X rays, mammograms, and CT scans. According to the American College of Radiology, radiologists overlook or misread evidence of disease about 30 percent of the time. Error rates are even higher for cancer—by some estimates, radiologists miss evidence of cancer 75 percent of the time on mammograms, and up to 90 percent of the time on chest X rays. In some cases, radiologists simply miss evidence that's in plain view because they're distracted or tired or overworked. The error rates are higher for some conditions. Sometimes—and this is more to the point for hospitalized patients—they see the evidence but draw the wrong conclusion.

Poor images also contribute to the problem. The film may be over- or underexposed, or the patient may be positioned in a way that hides the evidence.

Despite all of the advances in imaging technology, these error rates have changed little over the past fifty years. Nor does experience seem to matter: Studies show that error rates among experienced radiologists are almost identical to those of beginners.

Here are steps to reduce your risk of imaging misdiagnosis.

Don't take radiology reports as gospel. They're just one of many tools used for diagnosis. If they seem at odds with other evidence that your doctor has gathered, they might well be wrong.

When in doubt, ask for a second opinion. Ask your attending physician or specialist to have another radiologist review the films and make an independent judgment. (You shouldn't have to get another set made unless the image quality is too poor to interpret.) Evidence shows that having a second radiologist read the images can cut error rates approximately in half. If your doctor is reluctant, you can contact another radiologist yourself to arrange for a second opinion (check with your insurance company first to be sure they'll pay). Ask the radiology department to make a copy of the films and send them to the second radiologist. Ideally, the radiologist should be in a different practice so that the judgment is completely independent.

Ask your doctor whether he or she has spoken directly to the radiologist. Evidence shows that error rates are lower when radiologists have direct communication with the referring physician. Presumably it helps them get a better sense of what they're looking for.

Be sure the images are good. If the results come back inconclusive, encourage your doctor to find out whether the images were clear enough to make a good diagnosis, or whether they should be redone.

Find out whether the images ruled out disease or simply failed to show signs of disease. The first means that the disease definitely isn't there. The second means that it could be there and just didn't show up on the image.

Be Wary of Biopsies

A *biopsy* is a test in which a sample of tissue is removed from your body and sent to a laboratory for analysis. Most often used to diagnose or rule out cancer, biopsies have a reported error rate of between 1 and 5 percent. Those are pretty good odds—unless it happens to you. And the consequences of a missed diagnosis can be devastating.

The most common biopsy errors include:

- a benign (noncancerous) mass incorrectly judged to be malignant (cancerous)
- a malignant tumor incorrectly judged to be benign
- a malignant tumor correctly identified but staged improperly
- a tumor missed during the biopsy procedure—that is, the doctor removes healthy tissue instead
- the tissue sample prepared improperly, so that the laboratory can't see evidence of the tumor

A second, independent review of the sample can detect the first three of these errors, but not the last two. If the sample wasn't collected or prepared properly, the biopsy results may still appear normal. Therefore, *a "normal" biopsy result—even if confirmed—doesn't absolutely rule out cancer.* If other evidence still suggests the possibility of cancer, you may need to have the biopsy repeated.

17

Unnecessary Tests and Procedures

In the hospital, a *test* is any procedure performed to arrive at a diagnosis, monitor your condition, or find out whether your treatment is working. Unfortunately, tests are often ordered for none of these reasons. Doctors may order tests because they're "routine" or "just to be sure," because professional standards of care require them to perform certain tests based on your symptoms, or to protect themselves against malpractice suits.

RISK ALERT: GOOD INSURANCE COULD PUT YOU AT RISK

Beware if you have good insurance. Research suggests that old-fashioned "fee-for-service" insurance plans—which basically pay hospitals for anything the doctor orders—are more likely to result in unnecessary tests than HMOs and other managed-care plans. The reason is simple: If you have fee-for-service insurance, hospitals get paid for every test the doctor orders. In managed-care plans, they get a fixed amount from the insurance company for your hospital stay, no matter how many tests are ordered.

Ultimately, excessive testing reflects a common attitude in the health care system: the idea that a few extra tests might catch something and won't hurt anything other than the insurance companies' bottom line.

But unneeded tests are more than costly. They can be dangerous, for a number of reasons.

- Any procedure has some risk of injury or complication.
- The tests may produce false-positive results. That is, they may indicate that you have a medical problem that you don't really have—and therefore subject you to treatments you don't need. And these treatments, of course, come with their own risks.
- They may prolong your stay in the hospital while you're waiting to have the tests done or while you're waiting for the results. And the longer you're in the hospital, the greater the risk of complications.

To avoid unnecessary tests, ask the doctor to review with you what tests have been ordered and why each one is necessary. Tell him or her you'd prefer that testing be kept to a minimum—only if there's a clear reason for the test, rather than simply ordering a series of routine tests.

Redundant Tests

Redundant tests—tests that are repeated for no good reason—account for a large portion of unnecessary hospital tests. One study found that roughly one redundant test occurred for every twelve patients in the hospital. In other words, you have a one-in-twelve chance of receiving a redundant test during your hospital stay.

One reason for redundant tests is that so many tests are done. The same study found that each patient in the hospital received an average of 6.6 tests during his or her hospital stay.

Unnecessary Tests

In addition to redundant tests, you may be subjected to tests that you really don't need at all. Here are the most common unnecessary tests.

Digoxin Serum Levels

Digoxin is a widely used heart medication that helps strengthen the heartbeat, but it can be toxic if too much builds up in your bloodstream. So blood tests are used to measure these drug levels.

If you're receiving digoxin, ask the nurse how often digoxin serum levels are being tested. Though it's important to monitor these levels, doctors order these tests way too often in the hospital, says the AHCPR, a federal agency that studies the quality of medical care. The test should be used to set the right dosage at the beginning of therapy, with *occasional* follow-up testing to be sure the levels are holding steady—about once every three to ten days as long as everything is on track. (However, if the tests do show too much digoxin in your system, you'll be tested more often until the levels drop. With digoxin, there's a fine line between normal and too much.)

One study found, however, that many doctors routinely order *daily* testing of digoxin levels. In the vast majority of cases, these daily tests were completely unnecessary; they were just part of a battery of tests that the doctor ordered. (In about 8 percent of cases, the patient wasn't even taking the drug!) That can mean unnecessary needle sticks to draw blood or unnecessary handling of your IV line, both of which can increase your risk of infection.

ICU Tests

A variety of tests are common in the intensive care unit, including:

- blood gases
- glucose
- potassium levels
- electrocardiograms
- chest X rays

- sodium
- chloride
- complete blood count

Any or all of these tests may be necessary from time to time, but they tend to be ordered routinely and are frequently overused in the ICU. Of course, if you're critically ill, it's not usually the best time for you or your advocate to make an issue of overtesting. Rather, it's better to discuss the entire issue of tests with your doctor *before* you're admitted. Some doctors tend to be aggressive about ordering tests; others are less so. Be sure you're comfortable with your doctor's approach. And keep in mind that you have the right to refuse any test you don't want to have.

Strategies for Reducing Unnecessary Tests

- Talk to your doctors—especially your attending physician and any specialists—about tests *before* you need them. The best time to have this discussion is before you have to go into the hospital, if possible. Let your doctors know that you'd prefer to keep testing to a minimum. For example, you might say, "I understand that tests may be necessary, but I'd like to make sure I'm having them only if I really need them. What can we do to avoid unnecessary tests?"
- Ask why tests are being done and how they will affect your treatment. Sometimes the treatment will be the same regardless of the test results.

- Be sure your doctor knows what tests you've had recently, especially if you're being treated in the hospital by a specialist who hasn't treated you before. Often specialists haven't reviewed your entire medical history; they only know what's on your chart from the hospital. Keep a list of tests that you've recently had performed, so that you can check to be sure they're not ordered again.
- You can obtain a copy of all your test results. Keep them handy to give to your doctor.
- If you've undergone tests during a previous hospitalization or as an outpatient, make sure the results are made available to the physicians treating you in the hospital. (This may require a call to your primary-care physician, who's responsible for coordinating the specialists' care.) Similarly, if several specialists are treating you, be sure they all have access to your test results so that they don't order the same tests.
- Some doctors like to order a completely new set of tests just to reassure themselves. This is not an acceptable reason to subject you to more testing and expense. While you're in the hospital, know what tests have been ordered and what they're for. Your nurse can tell you.
- If you find yourself scheduled for tests you think you've already had, speak up! Question the nurse, doctor, or technician, especially if the test is uncomfortable or risky in any way (such as getting a duplicate set of X rays). If the only reason anyone can give you for having the test done again is "because the doctor ordered it," insist that they hold off until they can check why it's being ordered and whether it's really necessary.

18

Going Home

Just because you're getting out of the hospital doesn't mean you're out of the woods.

The final risk you face during your hospital stay is being released without a good discharge plan. Hospitals can't just wash their hands of you once your need for hospital care is done. They have a responsibility to develop a plan for your care after you leave. Written discharge plans are required by law for every hospitalized Medicare patient. Other insurers may require them as well. Whether required or not, *every patient should receive a discharge plan and written instructions before leaving the hospital.*

Just about every hospital has an office or department responsible for discharge planning. Usually nurses or social workers create the plans and review them with you.

But some hospitals do a better job than others. In some, discharge planning is little more than a formality—a few forms handed to you on your way out the door. In more enlightened hospitals, however, discharge planning is considered a key element of your hospital care. It begins when you're admitted and is an ongoing process.

Nurses, discharge planners, and quality assessment personnel should begin reviewing your chart during your stay to ensure that your recovery is on track and to identify what needs you might have when it's time to discharge you. They track your progress, look for complications, contact referral services, make extended-care arrangements, contact the home care nurses, check with your insurance company to find out what's covered, and assess your physical, emotional, and spiritual needs. Discharge planners work with the other departments such as pharmacy, nutrition, physical therapy, rehabilitation, and respiratory therapy.

During your stay, someone should be talking to you about what happens afterward. For example, will you have the help you need at home? If not, the discharge planner should be arranging for home-nursing care or other assistance. Will you need follow-up treatment, such as physical therapy or rehabilitation? Will it be done as an inpatient or an outpatient? Again, the discharge planner should be working with you to arrange this care and to find out what your insurance covers.

Your health care advocate can play an especially critical role in discharge planning. Often it's easier for the advocate to marshal the resources you need—for example, making arrangements for nursing care and the equipment you might need at home. And if necessary, the advocate can work with other loved ones and family members so they know what to expect when you're discharged and how they can help.

Major Risks

There are four key risks to avoid during discharge:

- being discharged too early
- being discharged to the wrong kind of aftercare
- not getting good instructions
- not having enough help at home

Discharged Too Early

How times have changed. Back in the old days, when hospitals got paid for every day you spent there, they were in no hurry to send you on your way. The longer you stayed, the more money they made.

But these days, many health plans pay hospitals a fixed fee for your care, whether you have to stay two days or twenty days. That means that the longer you stay, the more you cost the hospital. The incentives are exactly reversed: Now it's in the hospital's financial interest to get you in and out quickly.

That's not *necessarily* a bad thing. As we've seen, the less time you spend in the hospital, the less you're exposed to such risks as infection and medication errors. But if you're sent home too early, your recovery could be at risk.

How soon is too soon? The nursing staff should be evaluating you to be sure you're ready. But if you feel that you're going home too early, let your doctors and your nurses know. If you don't raise the issue, your caregivers may assume you're ready for discharge when you're not.

If you think you're being discharged too early, you

can challenge the decision. If you're a Medicare patient, for example, you'll be given a letter explaining how to appeal (see below). Other insurers may have similar procedures.

You have to appeal immediately, however. The hospital won't physically throw you out, but your insurer won't pay for you to stay once the doctor has determined you're ready to be discharged. You could be hit with a big hospital bill if you refuse to go.

Sample Medicare Discharge Form

NOTICE OF DISCHARGE & MEDICARE APPEAL RIGHTS

Enrollee's Name:_____

Date of Notice: _____

Health Insurance Claim (HIC) Number: _____

Admission Date: _____

Attending Physician: _____

Discharge Date: _____

Hospital: _____

Health Plan: _____

YOUR IMMEDIATE ATTENTION IS REQUIRED

Your doctor has reviewed your medical condition and has determined that you can be discharged from the Hospital because: [check one]

_____ You no longer require inpatient hospital care.

_____ You can safely get any medical care you need in another setting.

_____ Other (fill in the details) _____

This also means that, if you stay in the hospital, it is likely that your hospital charges for [*specify date of first noncovered day*] and thereafter will not be covered by your Health Plan.

The Hospital has developed a discharge plan which explains any follow-up care or medications you need. If you have questions about this follow-up care, you should discuss them with your doctor. If you have not received a discharge plan and wish to do so, please contact your nurse, social worker or doctor.

If you agree with your doctor's discharge decision, you can either read further to learn more about your appeal rights, or you can skip to the end of this notice and sign to show that you have received this notice.

However, if you disagree with your doctor's discharge decision, Medicare gives you the right to appeal. In that case, please continue reading to learn how to appeal a discharge decision, what happens when you appeal, and how much money you may owe.

IF YOU THINK YOU'RE BEING ASKED TO LEAVE THE HOSPITAL TOO SOON, REQUEST AN IMMEDIATE REVIEW.

HOW DO YOU GET AN IMMEDIATE REVIEW?

1. The [*Name of PRO*] is the name of the Peer Review Organization—sometimes called a PRO—authorized by Medicare to review the Hospital care provided to Medicare patients. **You or your authorized representative, attorney, or court appointed guardian** must contact the PRO by telephone or in writing: *[Name, address, telephone and fax number of the PRO].* If you file a written request, please write, **"I want an immediate review."**

2. **Your request must be made no later than noon of the first working day after you receive this notice.**

3. The PRO will make a decision within one full working day after it receives your request, your medical records, and any other information it needs to make a decision.

4. While you remain in the Hospital, your Health Plan will continue to be responsible for paying the costs of your stay until noon of the calendar day following the day the PRO notifies you of its official Medicare coverage decision.

WHAT IF THE PRO AGREES WITH YOUR DOCTOR'S DECISION DISCHARGE DECISION?

If the PRO agrees, you will be responsible for paying the cost of your Hospital stay beginning at noon of the calendar day following the day the PRO notifies you of its Medicare coverage decision.

WHAT IF THE PRO DISAGREES WITH YOUR DOCTOR'S DISCHARGE DECISION?

You will not be responsible for paying the cost of your additional Hospital days, except for certain convenience services or items not covered by your Health Plan.

WHAT IF YOU DON'T REQUEST AN IMMEDIATE REVIEW?

If you **remain** in the Hospital and do not request an immediate review by the PRO, you may be financially responsible for the cost of many of the services you receive beginning *[specify date of first noncovered day]*.

If you **leave** before *[specify date of first noncovered day]*, you will not be responsible for the cost of care. As with all hospitalizations, you may have to pay for certain convenience services or items not covered by your Health Plan.

WHAT IF YOU ARE LATE OR MISS THE DEADLINE TO FILE FOR AN IMMEDIATE REVIEW?

If you are late or miss the noon deadline to file for an immediate review by your PRO, you may still request an expedited (fast) appeal from your Health Plan. A "fast" appeal means your Health Plan will have to review your request within 72 hours. However, **you will not have automatic financial protection during the course of your appeal.** This means you could be responsible for paying the costs of your Hospital stay beginning *[specify date of first noncovered day]*.

HOW DO YOU REQUEST A FAST APPEAL?

You may call or fax your request to your Health Plan:

> Stamp or Print Here
> Name of Health Plan
> Address
> Phone # and Fax #

If you filed a request for immediate PRO review but were late in filing the request, the PRO will forward your request to your Health Plan as a request for a fast appeal.

If you're filing a written request, please write, "I want a fast appeal."

If you or any doctor asks your Health Plan to give you a fast appeal, your Health Plan must process your appeal within 72 hours of your request.

Your Health Plan may take up to 14 extra calendar days to make a decision if you request an extension or if your Health Plan can justify how the extra days will benefit you. For example, you should request an extension if you believe that you or your Health Plan need more time to gather additional medical information. Keep in mind that you may end up paying for this extended hospital stay.

Please sign to let us know you have received this notice of discharge and appeal rights. By signing this notice, you do not give up your right to appeal this discharge.

Signature of Medicare Enrollee or Authorized
Representative _____

Date _____

cc: [Health Plan]

The Wrong Kind of Aftercare

Keep in mind that going home isn't the only option. For example, you may be discharged to a rehab center, a skilled nursing facility, or a step-down unit (a unit of the hospital that provides less intensive nursing care) to complete your recovery. The discharge planner should work with you and your family to determine which kind of care is appropriate. Family support is a critical issue. You may be able to do your rehab as an outpatient if someone can drive you. If you're alone, you may be better off with an inpatient program.

If you need extended care, ask what choices you have. Is home care possible, or is another long-term care facility needed? Have a family member go and check out the facilities to be certain they can meet your needs in a safe environment.

Also confirm what your insurance or Medicare will pay for, and for how long. How long will you be expected to stay and what are your recovery goals? Who will be in charge of your care while the rehabilitation moves forward?

If you go to an extended-care facility, be sure you will be able to get a pass to go home with family members.

This is a good way for you to experience what it will be like getting around at home. Before going home, have your family or advocate inspect it for hazardous areas, such as loose carpets that could cause you to trip. Many rehabilitation programs will visit your home before you are discharged to evaluate the safety of your environment. You may want to consider some simple modifications at home to make it easier to get around, such as occupancy sensors that turn lights on automatically when you come into a room, and grab bars in the bathroom to make it easier to get in and out of the tub. Many of these modifications are inexpensive and can be done by anyone who's handy with tools. (For more information on these kinds of modifications—known as "universal design"—go to the Universal Design Web site at www.design.ncsu.edu/cud/.)

Discharged Without Instructions

A written discharge plan should be available for the most common types of illness and surgical patients. These plans can be tailored to your needs. You should have a copy of the plan.

You should also get a set of written instructions explaining how to care for yourself after you leave the hospital. They should include, for example, instructions on how to care for your surgical incision (if you have one), a list of your medications with dosage schedules, and any limitations on your activities, exercise, and nutrition.

If you haven't received such instructions, insist that they be provided to you in writing before you're discharged. You may not remember everything you've been told.

Written instructions often aren't enough. You will probably need discharge teaching as well to prepare you for going home. For example, a nurse, doctor, therapist, or technician should show you how to change your dressing or use any equipment that you'll need.

Not Enough Help at Home

It's dangerous to go home if there aren't people around to help you. If you live alone, or if your family isn't able to help you, let your doctor and nurses know, and be sure your discharge plan includes arrangements for nursing care or other assistance.

Critical Pathways

During your hospital stay, your nurses should be checking your recovery against guidelines known as *critical pathways*. These include basic self-care functions that you need to be able to perform before discharge. For example, if you will need to change your dressings or do certain exercises at home, these activities will be included in the pathways. Your nurses will check them off when they've confirmed that you can perform the tasks correctly. The pathway form becomes a part of your medical record.

At the very least, you should be able to perform your activities of daily living before you're discharged to home. These include getting out of bed, washing yourself, brushing your teeth, going to the toilet, dressing yourself, getting a glass of water, and getting to food and medicine. You may not be able to prepare your meals, but you should be able to feed yourself.

The pathways take into account a variety of factors—what disease or condition you have, your general health, whether you're going home or to another facility, how much family support is available, and so on. It's up to the doctor and nursing staff to determine what's appropriate for you and to tailor the discharge plan accordingly. You can't assume that a "standard" plan is safe for you.

For example, Nell had come into the hospital to have her appendix removed. The surgery went smoothly. She was discharged and told to make an appointment with the surgeon in four weeks.

But Nell didn't realize that she needed to change her dressing or care for her wound. Because she was obese, Nell couldn't see the incision area or reach it. Either nobody told her what she had to do, or she'd forgotten what she'd been told. She didn't receive written instructions or, if she did, she'd misplaced them.

By the time Nell arrived for her follow-up visit four weeks later, her incision was infected and was gaping open. She needed special dressings with medicated solution. By this time, it was obvious that Nell couldn't care for herself. She needed home-nursing care.

Yet despite these efforts, Nell's infection got worse, and she had to come back to the hospital for several weeks. If Nell had been more thoroughly assessed and educated before discharge, she probably could have avoided these complications.

Sylvia, seventy-six, lived alone. She suffered a stroke

affecting her right arm and leg. Admitted to the ICU, she was unable to walk, feed herself, or make any sense out of where she was. Gradually her strength and coordination started to return. When she was transferred to the regular medical floor, she thought she was home free. She started getting out of bed on her own and fell, scraping her arms, head, and legs.

Sylvia was transferred to the rehab unit for two weeks. All the nursing personnel and occupational therapists thought Sylvia was doing very well, and she was prepared for discharge.

Soon after she got home, Sylvia started doing some chores. She tripped and fell. Living alone and unable to get up, she lay for some hours before help arrived.

The next day, while Sylvia was walking with her cane, she lost control of her right leg and fell again. This time she fractured her pelvis. She was readmitted to the hospital and later was transferred to a nursing home for two months of physical rehabilitation.

Sylvia clearly was discharged too soon after her stroke, and it cost her a fractured pelvis. It wasn't safe for her to be at home alone. Yet, Sylvia told us later, she had a false sense of security when she was originally discharged, because everyone told her how well she was doing.

Making the Follow-up Appointment

It's surprising how many patients complicate their care because they don't get prompt follow-up care after they're discharged.

Be sure you have the phone number of your physician, the hospital, or other resources before you're discharged. If you've had surgery, arrange for your postoperative appointment before you leave the hospital if you can. Otherwise, call as soon as you can.

When you call, tell the receptionist that you're calling to make a posthospital office visit. Many times, patients call the doctor's office and are given an appointment for a date much later than the physician wanted. The secretary won't know you were in the hospital unless you tell her.

Again, this is a task that your advocate can help you with while you're recovering.

Strategies: A Checklist for Discharge

Here are some of the issues you should consider during the planning process.

- How will you get home? Will a family member drive you? Do you need a taxi? An ambulance?
- Will you be able to drive once you're home? If not, is a family member available to take you to appointments, shopping, and so on?
- How much and what kind of activity can you engage in? Can you, for example, walk the steps to the bedroom and bathroom? If not, do you need to rent a hospital bed and/or commode? Who pays?
- Can you shop for groceries? If not, can a family member help out, or do you need to arrange for meals on wheels?

- When do you need to see the doctor or therapist next? Has an appointment been set up?
- Will you be able to care for yourself—for example, can you change your own dressings? Do you need in-home nursing care? How often? And who pays?
- Do you have any special nutritional needs? Do you need supplements or special meals?
- When can you resume sexual activity?
- Do you know what drugs you're supposed to be taking? How often? Will your prescriptions be filled at the hospital before you leave, or do you have to get them filled on your own? Do you have medications at home that you were taking before you went into the hospital? Should you still be taking them? Do the dosages need to be adjusted?
- Do you know warning signs for any problems that may come up, and do you know what to do about them? For example, will you be able to recognize signs of infection in your surgical incision?
- Do you know what to do and whom to call in an emergency?
- Whom should you call if you have other questions after you get home?

Afterword: If You're Hurt

If you've been a victim of a medical error, what should you do about it?

The first, and often most difficult, step is to get your caregivers *to acknowledge that an error occurred.* If the mistake falls into a gray area—such as an infection that you might have gotten anyway—doctors and nurses may give themselves the benefit of the doubt rather than admit a mistake. They may even believe your injury was simply a case of bad luck and not due to anything they did. That's a dangerous attitude, because it means similar errors can happen again.

If your immediate caregivers won't acknowledge the error, you may want to take it further. You or your advocate can contact the nursing supervisor or the appropriate department head—for example, the head of the pharmacy if it was a medication error, or the chair of the infection control committee for infections.

Next, make sure that the doctor, nurses, and hospital have taken any necessary steps to limit damage from the mistake. Contact the hospital's risk management department and discuss your concerns with them.

In the Hospital

Be sure that the error is noted in your medical record. If you later decide to make a claim against the hospital, the medical record will be important evidence. Document for yourself the events of the error. Don't count on your medical record to be your best defense.

Before you're discharged, ask that you be sent an itemized copy of your bill, even if the insurance company is paying for it. Usually it takes about two weeks to get the bill after you're discharged. Were you charged to treat a problem that the hospital itself caused? For example, did you have to spend extra days in the hospital for treatment? Undergo additional tests? If so, talk to the risk management department and ask that the hospital remove those charges (but save a copy of both versions of the bill).

The hospital may refuse to make an adjustment, especially if your insurance company is paying the bill. If so, send a letter to the insurance company explaining what happened and recommending that it investigate the charges and the care you received. Send a copy to the hospital and keep a copy for yourself. The insurance company will probably pay the charges anyway—but you've helped create a paper trail documenting the medical error. That will be important if you decide to make a claim later.

If you're responsible for paying part of the bill, talk to the hospital. Many times, it will discount your out-of-pocket portion if the charges resulted from a medical error.

No Harm, No Foul?

Most medical errors don't result in significant injuries. If you miss a medication or take the wrong pill or get an unnecessary test, usually no physical harm is done as long as it's an isolated incident.

That's the key question: Was it an isolated incident? Or the tip of the iceberg? Hospitals will never eliminate every error. There are just too many things going on, and too many unknowns.

But some errors reflect a *systems* breakdown. And if the system isn't fixed, the same errors will keep happening again—and could happen to you again.

Beware of the "Snowball Effect"

Errors tend to snowball. When serious injuries occur, it's often because several things went wrong. In hindsight, it's often possible to identify any number of points in the process where somebody could—and should—have called a time-out.

Often, caregivers miss the big picture. They see a series of small incidents, each manageable on its own, but they don't connect the dots and see how these mistakes compound one another.

If you (or your advocate) see errors starting to snowball, try to create a time-out for everyone to assess the situation. Ask the nurse to call the doctor. Or ask tough questions to make everybody take a step back and take a second look at the situation. For example:

- Why did this error occur?
- Who was involved?
- Could it happen again?
- What's been done to prevent it from happening again?
- What could happen as a result of this error? What *else?* (Often people consider only the most likely possibilities, not all of the possibilities.)
- What's being done to prevent or manage those problems?
- Does the nursing supervisor know what happened? Does the doctor?
- Has the risk manager been notified of the error?

If you think these questions sound a little confrontational, you're right. The goal isn't to prosecute the person who made the error but to be sure everyone is paying enough attention to it.

If you've been the victim of a medical error, you or your advocate may want to get in touch with the risk manager. Every reputable health facility has a risk management department. Its job is to enforce and monitor safety in the workplace for employees and patients. Talk to the risk manager after the injury and discuss where the error occurred and what allowed the incident to occur. (But keep in mind that not all incidents are brought to the attention of the risk management department.) Ask what steps are being taken to avoid similar incidents in the future.

The risk management department also keeps records of incidents to help improve hospital policy, prevent further incidents, and keep a legal record. This information is available to you and your lawyer. Your lawyer may need to ask for some records.

At the time of the incident, be sure an incident report form is filled out by those involved. It documents the event. The incident report is not a permanent part of your medical record but is kept in the risk management office. This is a valuable piece of information if you have to file a claim later.

Find out who was involved in the incident: physicians, nurses, physical therapists, radiologists, and so on. Get as much in writing as you can. If you are told you won't have to pay for the stitches you had put in as a result of your fall, be sure you have that in writing and signed by the risk manager or others in authority. Ask what hospital policy is in the event of an injury. Again, get it in writing.

When You Get Home

Follow your doctor's orders and document any problems you have with written notes. Do not rely on your memory.

If you've been injured, show someone the injury or have a photo taken so you have witnesses or evidence later.

If you notice a problem from an injury after you get home, notify your doctor, call the risk management department of the hospital, and notify the department director of the nursing floor you were on. Keep everyone well informed of events so there are no surprises. If you require nursing visits at home, be sure the nurse documents the visit and the reasons for it. You have a right to read these notes.

Should You Sue?

The vast majority of medical errors never result in a lawsuit. Many errors go undetected. Or even if the nurses or doctor think they made a mistake, they may not tell you about it.

Also, medical malpractice lawsuits are lengthy, difficult, and expensive. Since most malpractice lawyers work on contingency—they don't get paid unless they win—many won't take a case unless the injuries are severe and the hospital's liability is clear. As one malpractice attorney said, "If the patient can walk into our office, we're not likely to take the case." Not every lawyer goes to that extreme, but most choose their cases carefully.

When lawsuits do go to trial, patients win only about half the time. One reason is that malpractice suits are judged by a different standard than ordinary negligence lawsuits. It's not enough to show that nurses or doctors caused your injury, or even to show that they were negligent. You have to show that they failed to meet a "reasonable standard of care," which is basically defined as what their professional peers would do in a similar situation.

Another critical element is damages—how much harm was done, and what is it worth in dollars and cents? If the hospital made a mistake but you didn't suffer any serious harm, it is difficult to collect damages.

The legal notions of damages may not be what you expect. First, the courts look at *economic* damages—what did the error cost you? Your medical bills are part of that equation, although if your insurance company already paid them, it may be entitled to those winnings, not you. Another part of economic damages involves your ability to earn a living. From an economic standpoint, the courts have concluded that while all men are created equal, some lives are worth more than others. If a medical error kills an eighty-two-year-old widower who was already seriously ill, the economic damages are little if any: He wasn't working, and his life expectancy was short anyway. If a similar error kills an infant, the loss-of-income damages are likely to be far higher, since the infant was deprived of an entire lifetime of earning capacity.

Damages also include the costs for any long-term or permanent care you require as a result of any disability, such as skilled nursing care. That can lead to another bizarre outcome: Often a hospital pays less if a patient dies than if the patient is only injured.

On top of these costs, courts often award *noneconomic* damages, such as compensation for pain and suffering or loss of consortium (your spouse's loss of your companionship). In some states, noneconomic damages have a dollar limit. Some argue that these caps are unfair to patients who are catastrophically injured and may endure a lifetime of suffering.

All that being said, many malpractice lawsuits are filed and won every year (or, more accurately, most are settled before going to court). So if you feel you were the victim of medical negligence and suffered serious harm, it may be worth consulting an attorney.

The consultation is usually free, and you won't pay anything out of pocket if the lawyer agrees to take the case. If you lose, you owe the lawyer nothing. If you win or the case is settled, the lawyer will take a hefty cut—typically about 40 percent.

Be wary about trying to settle the case on your own without an attorney. Even if the hospital does offer to settle, you may be selling yourself short.

Don't sign any releases, waivers, or settlement offers until you've had a lawyer look them over. Even if you don't think you suffered any serious harm, don't sign anything. Otherwise you may not be able to make a claim later if further problems develop. And don't worry that the hospital will somehow retaliate against you if you refuse to sign: Faced with a potential lawsuit, the last thing the hospital wants to do is add insult to injury.

Resources

If you want to find out more about your disease or condition, the treatments available, and the risks, there's a vast amount of information available on the Internet, at the bookstore, and at libraries (both public and medical libraries).

All that information is something of a two-edged sword, however. For one thing, a lot of it is inaccurate. That's especially true on the Internet, where anybody can put up just about any kind of information whether it's true or not. Especially when you're dealing with serious diseases such as cancer, you have to be careful on the Net: It's a great place for charlatans and con artists to take advantage of desperate people.

To be safe, stick with sources that are well known and well respected. Use published Web sites from universities, public health sites, and medical journals, and sites that are sponsored or endorsed by major health associations such as the American Heart Association (www.american-heart.org), the Arthritis Foundation (www.arthritis.org), and the American Cancer Society (www.cancer.org). These sites have links to other reputable sites for more information. Be wary of any Web site that has a commercial purpose—whether it's to promote a "secret cure," an exclusive clinic, or a malpractice attorney—or that urges you to buy something or call for more information.

Another way to be sure that sources are on the up-and-up: Look at the sources *they* cite. If they don't cite sources, it probably means you're dealing with someone's unsupported opinion.

Also check to see if more than one reputable source is saying the same thing. Consensus is important when weighing opinions and making decisions.

Even when information is accurate, it's often hard to understand. The National Library of Medicine's (NLM) Web site (www.nlm.nih.gov), for example, allows you to search its vast database of medical journal articles, the same database used by top medical researchers. (And it's free, courtesy of your federal government.) But unless you know how to search—and how to sift through the dense scientific language—you're likely to be overwhelmed.

In this section, we offer some resources that can get you started, from leading health organizations and other trustworthy sources. Most were created with consumers in mind and offer useful advice in plain English.

If you want to delve further, it may be useful to find a medically knowledgeable guide—for example, a nurse, medical librarian, or someone else who can help you zero in on the information you need *and* help you understand what it means. If you find a willing medical librarian or researcher, you can ask him or her to help you search the NLM site for *review* articles pertaining to your disease or condition. These articles, written by experts for practicing physicians, give you an overview of recent advances and treatment controversies. Though they may be slow going, the key points are usually understandable to lay readers.

Patient organizations, support groups, and self-help groups are also a good source for finding people who've been down the road before you and can help guide your way.

And, of course, your doctors should be your first, last, and best consultants to answer your questions, help guide your research, and put you in touch with reputable self-help groups and other resources.

Here are some resources that can get you started. (Note: Web sites come and go, and some of these links may no longer be current. Search engines, such as Google, AltaVista, and Excite, can help you find updated links if they're available.)

Anesthesia

Free booklets on what you should know about anesthesia are available from the American Society of Anesthesiologists, 520 North Northwest Highway, Park Ridge, IL 60068-2573, (847) 825-5586; and the American Association of Nurse Anesthetists, 222 South Prospect Avenue, Park Ridge, IL 60068-4001, (847) 692-7050.

Cancer

"Talking With Your Doctor" focuses on a healthy doctor-patient relationship and suggests questions for patients to ask their doctor. It's written for cancer patients but is also helpful to others. It's free from the American Cancer Society, 1-800-ACS-2345, www.cancer.org.

Choosing a Doctor

"Health Care's Front Line: Primary Care Physicians" discusses choosing a primary care doctor and making the most of the first visit. This resource is part of a series published by the Health Pages' on-line magazine. The Web site is www.thehealthpages.com.

Clinical Practice Guidelines

Clinical practice guidelines are developed by groups of experts and describe their consensus on the best practices in medicine. The National Guideline Clearinghouse makes clinical practice guidelines available to the public via the Web. The clearinghouse was developed by the American Medical Association and the American Association of Health Plans. The guidelines tend to be technical. The Web site is www.guideline.gov.

Clinical Trials

"Taking Part in Clinical Trials: What Cancer Patients Need to Know" is a booklet by the National Cancer Institute describing how clinical trials work and their possible benefits and drawbacks. It's free from Cancer Information Service, 1-800-4-CANCER (1-800-422-6237), 9:00 A.M.–4:30 P.M. EST. You can also go to the Clinical Trials Web site at www.cancer.gov/clinicaltrials.

Hospitals and Nursing Homes

HospitalSelect is an on-line hospital locator that has basic information on all U.S. hospitals: size, capabilities, accreditation. The site also has links to the American Medical Association home page that lists physicians and specialists: www.ama-assn.org.

The Web site of the Joint Commission on Accreditation of Healthcare Organizations offers detailed information on the quality of individual hospitals. Go to www.jcaho.org.

A copy of the patient's bill of rights—which spells out what you can expect from a hospital—is available for free from the American Hospital Association: (312) 422-3000. Or go to www.aha.org. Click on Resource Center; under Advisories click on "Patient's Bill of Rights."

"All Hospitals Are Not Created Equal" is an on-line resource that provides information and questions to ask to help you choose the hospital that best suits your needs. It's part of a series published by Health Pages' on-line magazine. The Web site is www.thehealthpages.com/articles/ ar-hosps.html.

"Choosing a Hospital and Hospital Quality Checklist" is a Web site offered by the Pacific Business Group on Health: www.healthscope.org/hospital/default.asp.

Healthfinder is a government-sponsored site that provides a gateway to reliable consumer health information from the federal government and other organizations: www.healthfinder.gov.

Living Wills and Medical Powers of Attorney

The Web site www.nolo.com offers extensive information on these and other legal issues.

Medical Treatments

The "FDA Guide to Choosing Medical Treatments" is designed to help consumers avoid fraud and deception when choosing medical treatment. Order Reprint 95-1223 free from the Food and Drug Administration, Office of Consumer Inquiries: HFE-88, 5600 Fishers Lane, Rockville, MD 20857, (301) 443-3170. The Web site is www.fda.gov.

Medications

"Prescription Medicines and You" is available free from the Agency for Health Care Policy and Research and the National Council on Patient Information and Education. It includes tips for getting involved in your treatment, asking the right questions about your prescriptions, and keeping track of your medicines. The Web site is www.ahrq.gov/consumer/ncpiebro.htm.

Pain Control After Surgery

"Pain Control After Surgery: A Patient's Guide" is available free from the Agency for Health Care Policy and Research. For a copy of this consumer version of the AHCPR-supported clinical practice guideline and for information on other patient guides, write to AHCPR Publications Clearinghouse, P.O. Box 8547, Silver Spring, MD 20907, or call 1-800-358-9295.

Personal Health History

A confidential form that you can fill out and use to track your health and medicine history is on the American Medical Association Web site: www.ama-assn.org. Select Search, and enter "personal health history."

Second Opinions

For a free brochure on "Medicare Coverage for Second Surgical Opinions: Your Choice Facing Elective Surgery," write to Health Care Financing Administration, Publications, NI-26-27, 7500 Security Boulevard, Baltimore, MD 21244-1850. Ask for Publication #HCFA 02173.

To get the name of a specialist in your area who can give you a second opinion, ask your primary doctor or surgeon, the local medical society, or your health insurance company. Medicare beneficiaries may also obtain information from the U.S. Department of Health and Human Services' Medicare hotline: 1-800-638-6833.

Specific Diseases or Conditions

For almost every disease, there is a national or local association or society that publishes consumer information. Check your local telephone directory. There are also organized groups of patients with certain illnesses that can often provide information about a condition, alternative treatments, and experience with local doctors and hospitals. Ask your hospital or doctors if they know of any patient groups related to your condition. Also, your local public library has medical reference materials about health care treatments.

For further information, consult *The Savvy Patient: How to Be an Active Participant in Your Medical Care* by

David R. Stutz, M.D., and Bernard Feder, Ph.D. (Consumer Reports Books, 1990).

Information about women's health, men's health, and treatments for arthritis, diabetes, and other conditions is available from the Health Pages' on-line magazine. The Web site is www.thehealthpages.com.

Support Groups

Self-help or support groups offer support to people with disabilities, cancer, and many other health problems. The groups are made up of people who have "been there" and who share experiences and information. Call the American Self-Help Clearinghouse for information on national groups. It also can refer you to any state or local self-help clearinghouses in your area. If you want to start your own self-help group, the clearinghouse has information to help you. Call (973) 625-3037 (or from New Jersey only, 1-800-367-6274), or write to American Self-Help Clearinghouse, St. Clare's Health Services, 25 Pocono Road, Denville, NJ 07834-2995. On the Internet, go to the site www.mentalhelp.net/selfhelp.

Surgery

The American College of Surgeons (ACS) has a free series of pamphlets on "When You Need an Operation."

These documents are available on-line at www.facs.org/
public_info/ppserv.html. For print copies, write to the
ACS, Office of Public Information, 633 N. Saint Clair
Street, Chicago IL 60611. Topics in this series range from
general information about surgery to specific surgical procedures.

Talking with Your Doctor

"Talking With Your Doctor: A Guide for Older People"
suggests ways to discuss health concerns, medicines, and
issues important to older people. It's free from the
National Institute on Aging Information Center, Building
31, Room 5C27, 31 Center Drive MSC 2292, Bethesda,
MD 20892-2292, (301) 496-1752, TTY 1-800-222-
4225. The Web site is www.nih.gov/nia.

The Family Practice Health Site sponsored by the
American Association of Family Physicians contains a
wealth of information for you and your family. The Web
site is www.familydoctor.org.

Bibliography

Bades, D. "Preventing Surgical Errors and Adverse Events Using Information Technology." Program abstract from American College of Surgeons 88th Clinical Congress, Nov. 1–4, 2002, Philadelphia, PA.

Barclay, L. "Hospitals Make Medication Errors in 19% of Doses." *Archives of Internal Medicine* 162 (Sept. 2000): 1897–1903.

———. "Preventable Medical Errors: A News Maker Interview with Robert J. Blendon." *New England Journal of Medicine* 347(24) (2002): 1933–40, 2965–67.

Bartlett, D., and Davidhizar, R. "What Scares Patients About the Hospital." *Health Care Supervisor* 13(1) (Sept. 1994): 47–52.

Beckerman, A., Grossman, D., and Marquez, L. "Cardiac Catheterization: The Patients' Perspective." *Heart and Lung* 24(3) (May–June 1995): 213–9.

Behrns, K. *Patient Safety: Methods to Assess Risk and Improve Outcomes.* American College of Surgeons 88th Clinical Congress. Nov 1–4, 2002, Philadelphia, PA.

Bond, C. A., Raul, C. L., and Franke, T. "Clinical Pharmacy Services, Hospital Pharmacy Staffing and Medication Errors in United States Hospitals." *Pharmacotherapy* 22(2) (Feb. 2002): 134–147.

Braunschweig, C., Gomez, S., and Sheean, P. M. "Impact of Declines in Nutritional Status on Outcomes in Adult Patients Hospitalized for More than 7 Days." *Journal of the American Dietetic Association* 100(11) (Nov. 2000): 1316–24.

Bussing, A. "Stress and Burnout in Nursing: Studies in Different Work Structures and Work Schedules." Congress on Occupational Health. *Occupational Health for Health Care Workers* (1993): 399–405.

Colby, P. "Missing the Train." *Connecticut Nursing News* 71(2) (Jun.–Aug.): 1, 4.

Conley, D., Schultz, A. A., and Selvin, R. "The Challenge of Predicting Patients at Risk for Falling: Development of the Conley Scale." *MedSurg Nursing* 8(6) (Dec. 1999): 348–54.

Dennis, K. "Patient's Control and the Information Imperative: Clarification and Confirmation." *Nursing Research* 39(3) (May–June 1990): 162–66.

Fields, W. L., and Loveridge, C. "Critical Thinking and Fatigue: How Do Nurses on 8 and 12 Hour Shifts Compare." *Nursing Economics* 6(1988): 189–91.

Forrester, D. A., McCabe-Bender, J., and Tiedeken, K. "Fall Risk Assessment of Hospitalized Adults and

Follow-up Study." *Journal for Nurses in Staff Development* 15(6) (Nov.–Dec. 1999): 251–9.

Glauser, M., et al. *Global Antibiotic Resistance in the Hospital Setting: Trends, Impacts, and Successful Interventions for the Prevention and Management of Outbreaks.* University of Kentucky Office of Continuing Medical Education, Dec. 2000.

Hart, D., and Bossert, E. "Self-Reported Fears of Hospitalized School-Age Children." *Journal of Pediatric Nursing* 9(2) (April 1994): 83–90.

Hart, S. "Wards of Fear." *Nursing Times* 94(17) (Apr. 29–May 5, 1998): 28–9.

Horsley, J. "When Is a Shift Too Long to Be Safe?" *RN* 57(10) (Oct. 1994): 76,78.

Hupcey, J. E., Penrod, J., and Morse, J. M. "Establishing and Maintaining Trust During Acute Care Hospitalizations." *Scholarly Inquiry for Nursing Practice* 14(3) (Fall 2000): 227–42.

Lacy, M., Ellenberger, J., Rehwaldt, M., and Theobald, D. "How to Quell Families' Fears." *Contemporary Longterm Care* 15(3) (March 1992): 26, 85.

O'Sullivan, A. "President's Message: Staffing for Safe Care." *Illinois Nurses Association, Chart* 98(2) (Mar.–Apr. 2001): 2.

Poissonnet, C. M., and Veron, M. "Health Effects of Work Schedules in Healthcare Professions." *Journal of Clinical Nursing* 9(1) (Jan. 2000): 13–23.

Pollman, L., and Moog, R. "Differences in Shift Work Tolerance in Hospital Employees." Congress on Occupational Health. *Occupational Health for Health Care Workers* (1993): 79–83.

"Report Confirms Nursing Shortage." *Journal of Psychosocial Nursing and Mental Health Services.* 39(5) (May 2001): 9.

Rock, A. "How Hospitals Are Gambling with Your Life." *Reader's Digest* (Sept. 2001): 252–68.

Rutledge, D. N., Donaldson, N. E., and Pravikoff, D. S. "Fall Risk Assessment and Prevention in Healthcare Facilities." *Online Journal of Clinical Innovations* 1(9) (Dec. 15, 1998): 1–33.

Sakalys, J. "The Political Role of Illness Narratives." *Journal of Advanced Nursing* 31(6) (2000): 1469–75.

Schneider, P. J. "Applying Human Factors in Improving Medication Use Safety." *American Journal of Health-System Pharmacy* 59(12) (Sept. 2002): 1155–59.

Scrimshaw, N. S., and SanGiovanni, J. P. "Synergism of Nutrition, Infection, and Immunity: An Overview." *American Journal of Clinical Nutrition* 66(2) (Aug. 1994): 464S–77S.

Shafer, A., et al. "Preoperative Anxiety and Fear: A Comparison of Assessments by Patients and Anesthesia and Surgery Residents." *Anesthesia Analogues* 83(6) (Dec. 1996): 1285–91.

Spong, F. W. "A Hospital's No Place for a Sick Person." *Medical Economics* 75(8) (Apr. 27, 1998): 140, 143–4.

Wakefield, M. K. "Health Policy and Politics. Hard Numbers, Hard Choices: Seeking Solutions to the Nursing Shortage." *Nursing Economics* 19(2) (Mar.–Apr. 2001): 80–1.

Warren, J., Holloway, I., and Smith, P. "Fitting In: Maintaining a Sense of Self During Hospitalization." 37(3) (2000): 229–35.

Washburn, M. S. "Fatigue and Critical Thinking on

Eight and Twelve Hour Shifts." *Nursing Management* 22(9) (Sept. 1991): 80A-CC, 80D-CC.

Whitney, S. L., and Rossi, M. M. "Falls and Balance Issues in Long-Term Care." *Topics in Geriatric Rehabilitation* 15(2) (Dec. 1999): 1–13.

"Why Patients Complain and What Health Professionals Can Do About It." *Strategic Health Excellence* 13(4) (Apr. 2000): 11–20.

Wolfgang, A. P. "Job Stress in the Health Professions: A Study of Physicians, Nurses and Pharmacists." *Behavioral Medicine* (1988): 14, 43–7.

Wunderink, R., et. al. *The Importance of Gram-Positive Bacterial Infections in the Hospital Setting.* Symposium, American College of Chest Physicians (2002). Philadelphia, PA.

Index

About the Authors

Gail Van Kanegan, R.N., M.S.N., C.N.P., is a certified advanced practice nurse with thirty years' experience in the medical field. Her career as a nurse has taken her through the emergency room, obstetric department, medical surgical floors, intensive care, cardiac care, and the cardiology department of major hospitals. During the last six years she has been a family nurse practitioner, providing primary care to patients. The focus of her practice is to help the patients learn about diseases, understand the options for care, prevent health problems, and become as healthy as possible. Gail is a public speaker for health care issues nationally and throughout Illinois, speaking to professionals and consumers. She is an advocate for the public to learn their health care rights and regularly writes articles on consumer health care issues.

Michael Boyette is a veteran medical journalist and has written six consumer-health books. He was also editor-in-chief of *Hospital Risk Control,* one of the pioneering publications in the field of hospital risk management and quality assurance. He has written more than a hundred in-depth articles on all aspects of hospital safety and mal-practice, ranging from patient falls to medication errors to surgical mishaps. This background gives him a behind-the-scenes understanding of hospitals, what can go wrong in them, and how patients can protect themselves.